Contents

Trace the lines

Trace the shapes

Trace the letters

Trace the numbers

Trace and match

Connect the dots

Symmetry drawing

Shadow matching

Item hunt

Coloring pages

Continue the pattern

Eye-hand coordination

Spot differences

Mazes

Word scramble

Telling time

Sudoku

Find two same pictures

Trace the lines

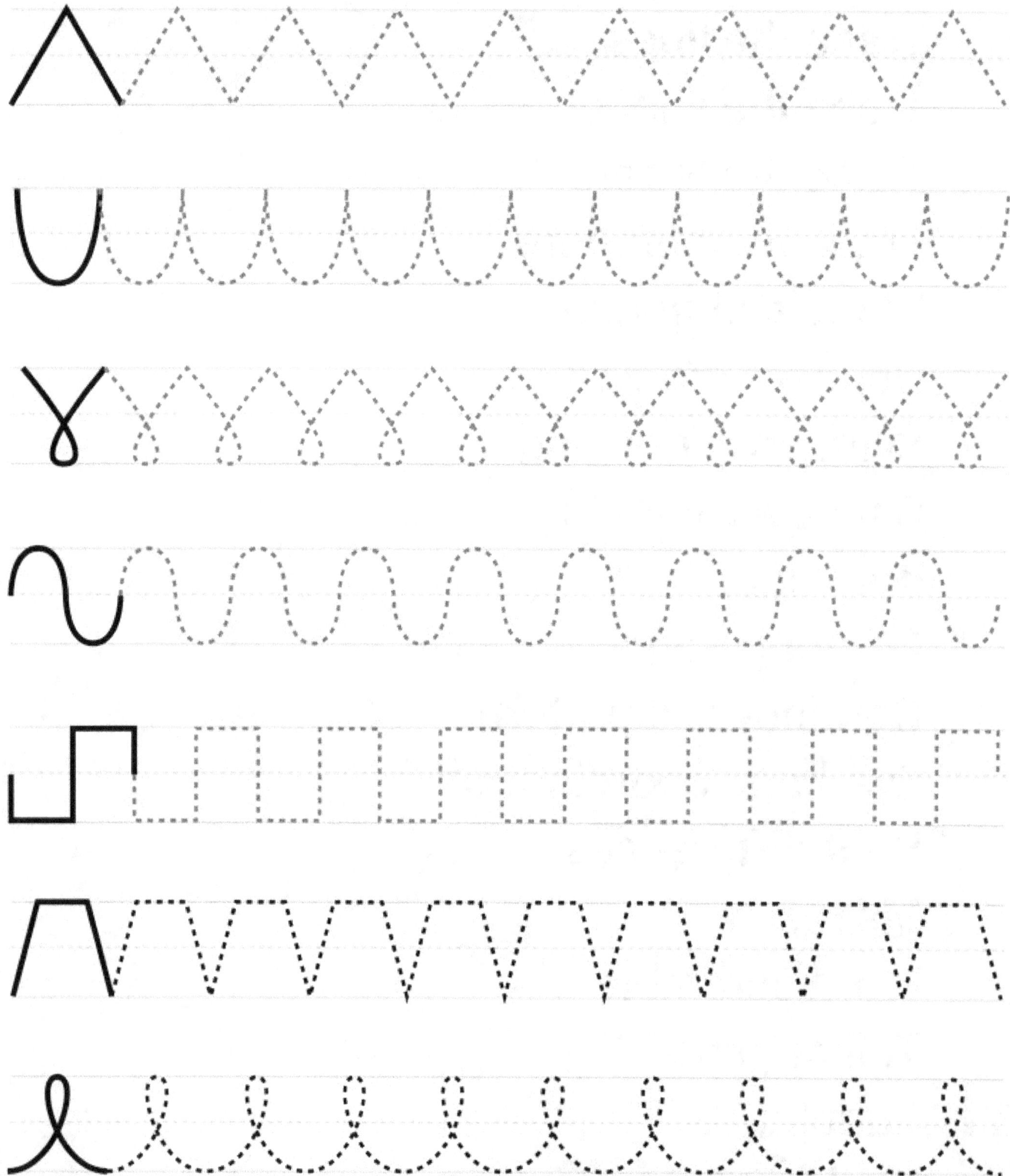

Trace the lines

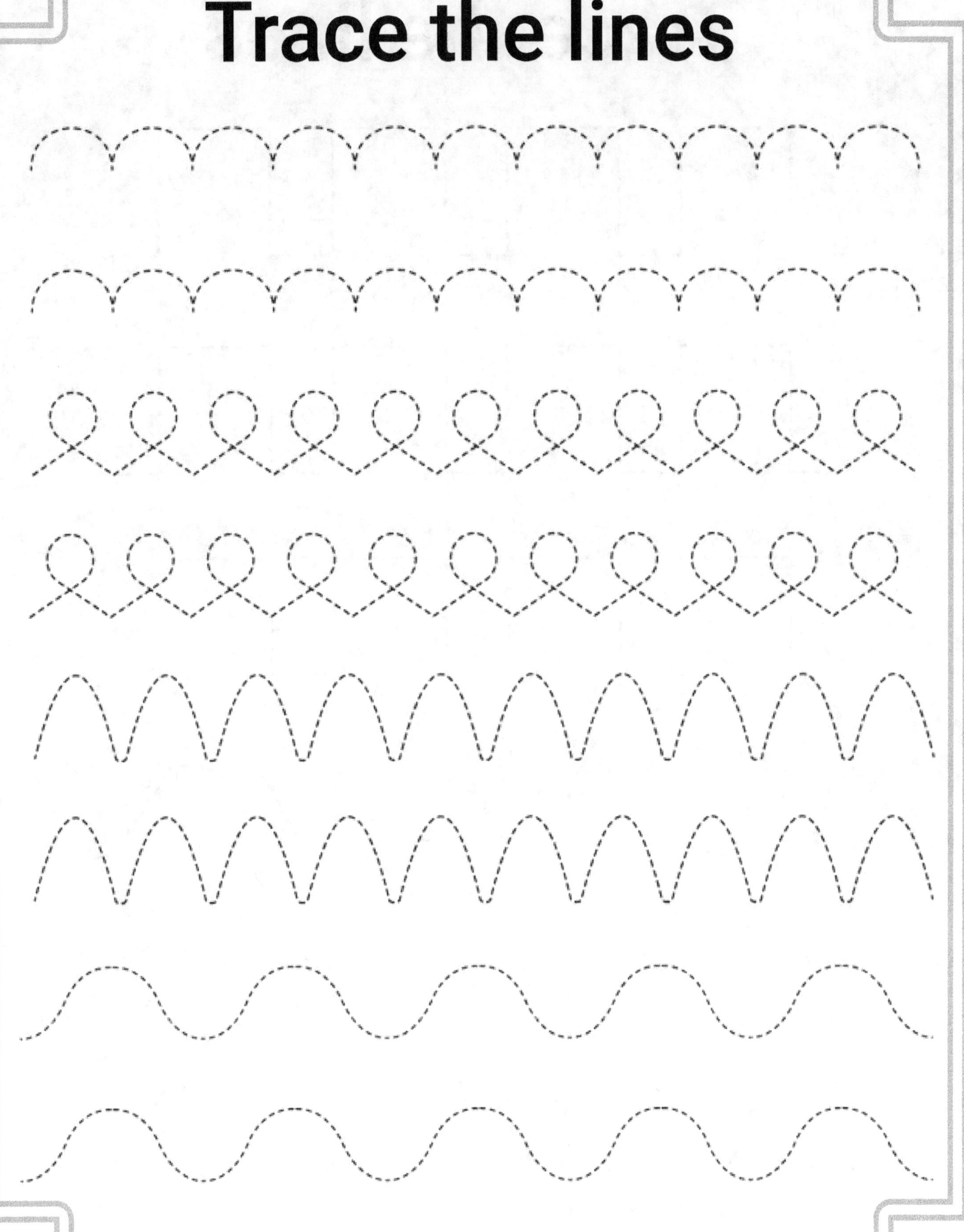

Trace the lines

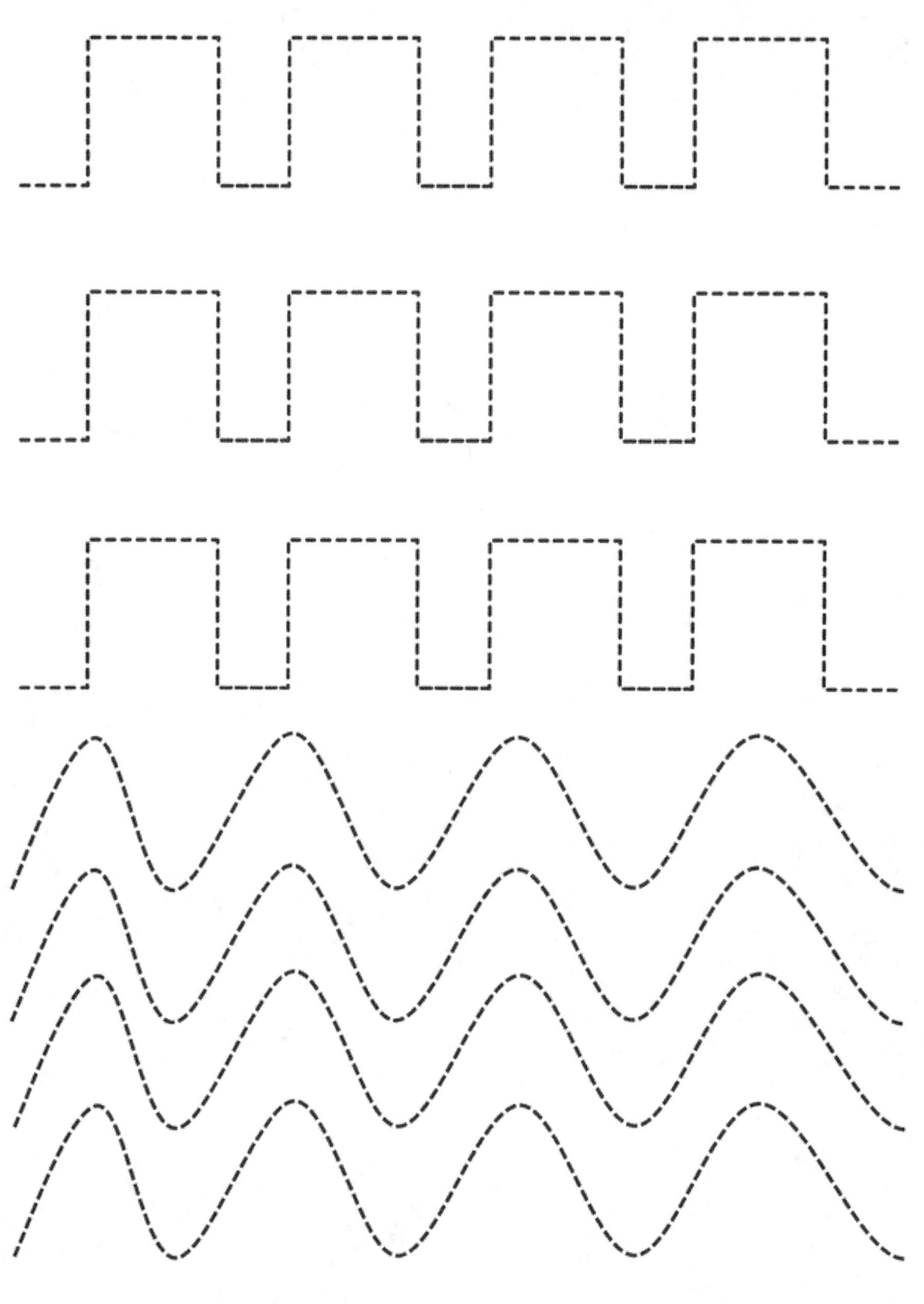

Trace the shapes

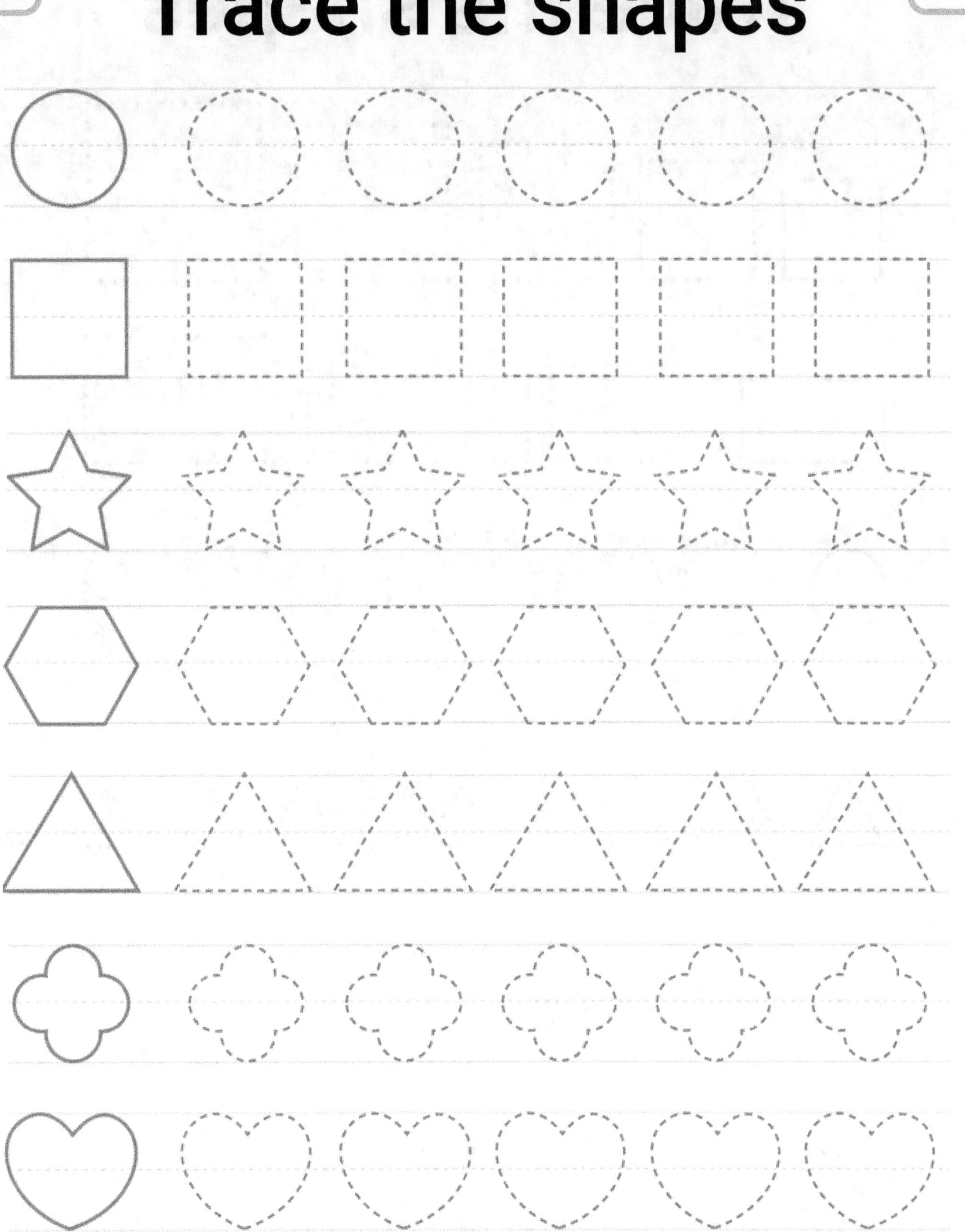

Trace the shapes

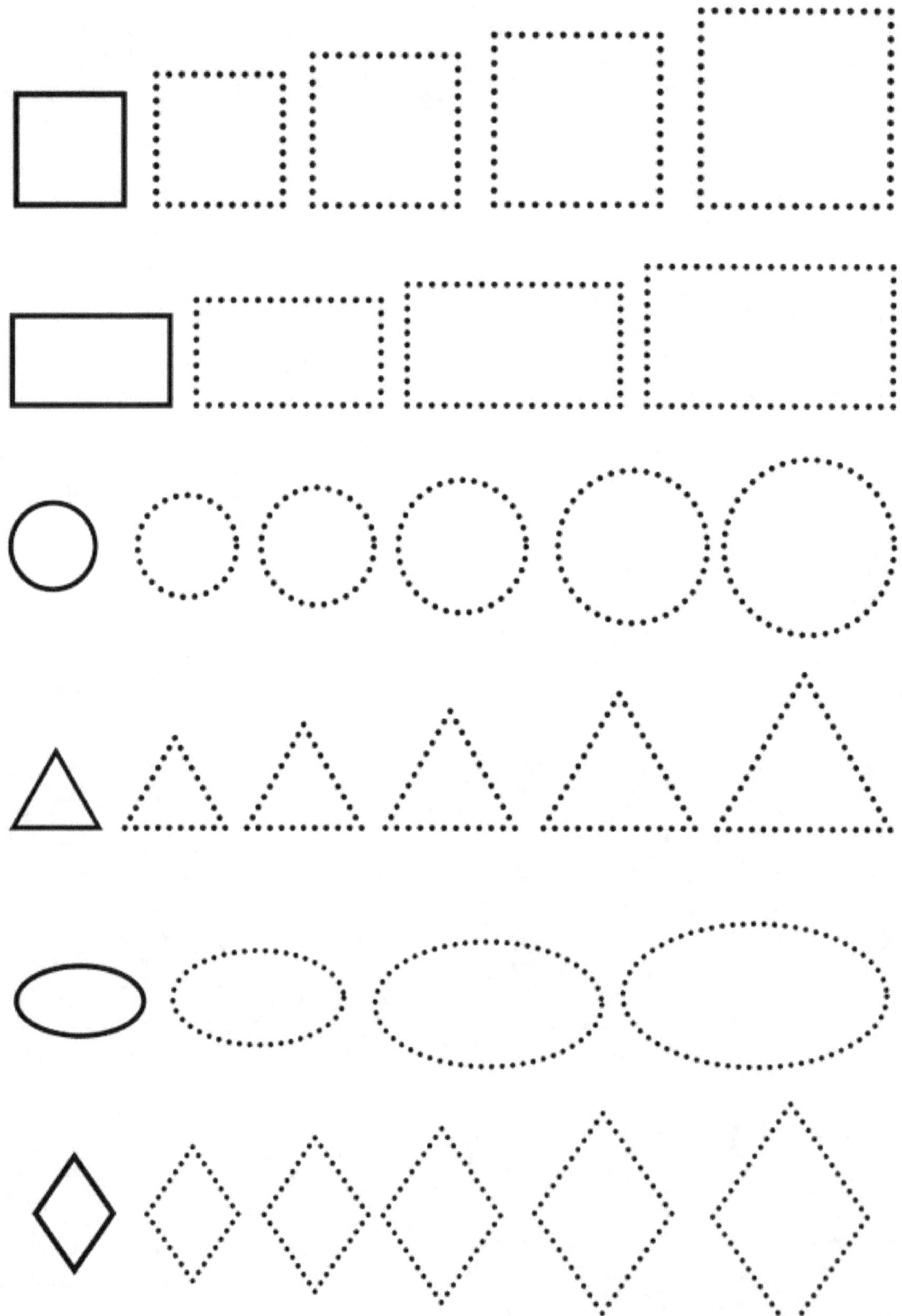

Trace the shapes

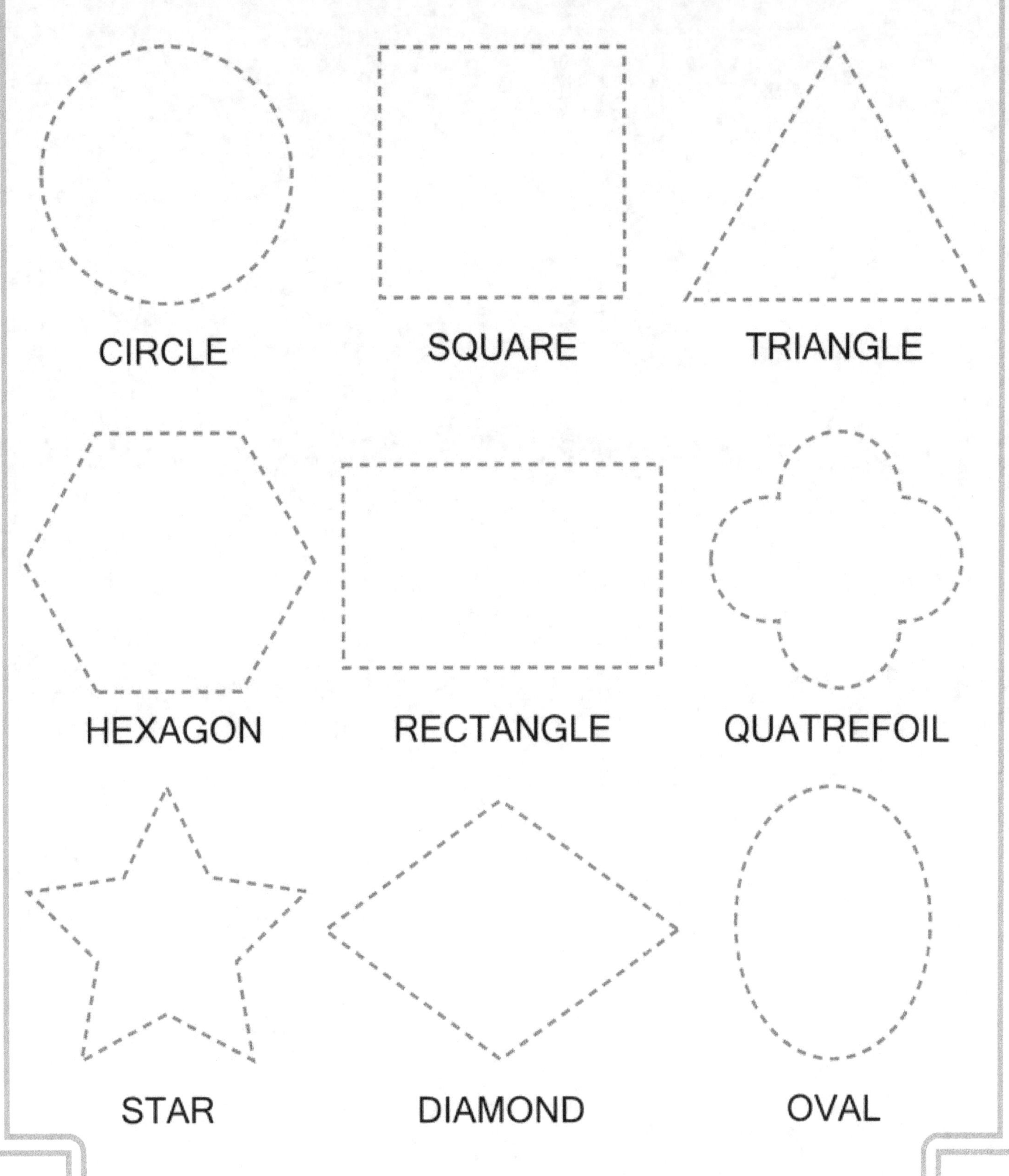

Trace the letters

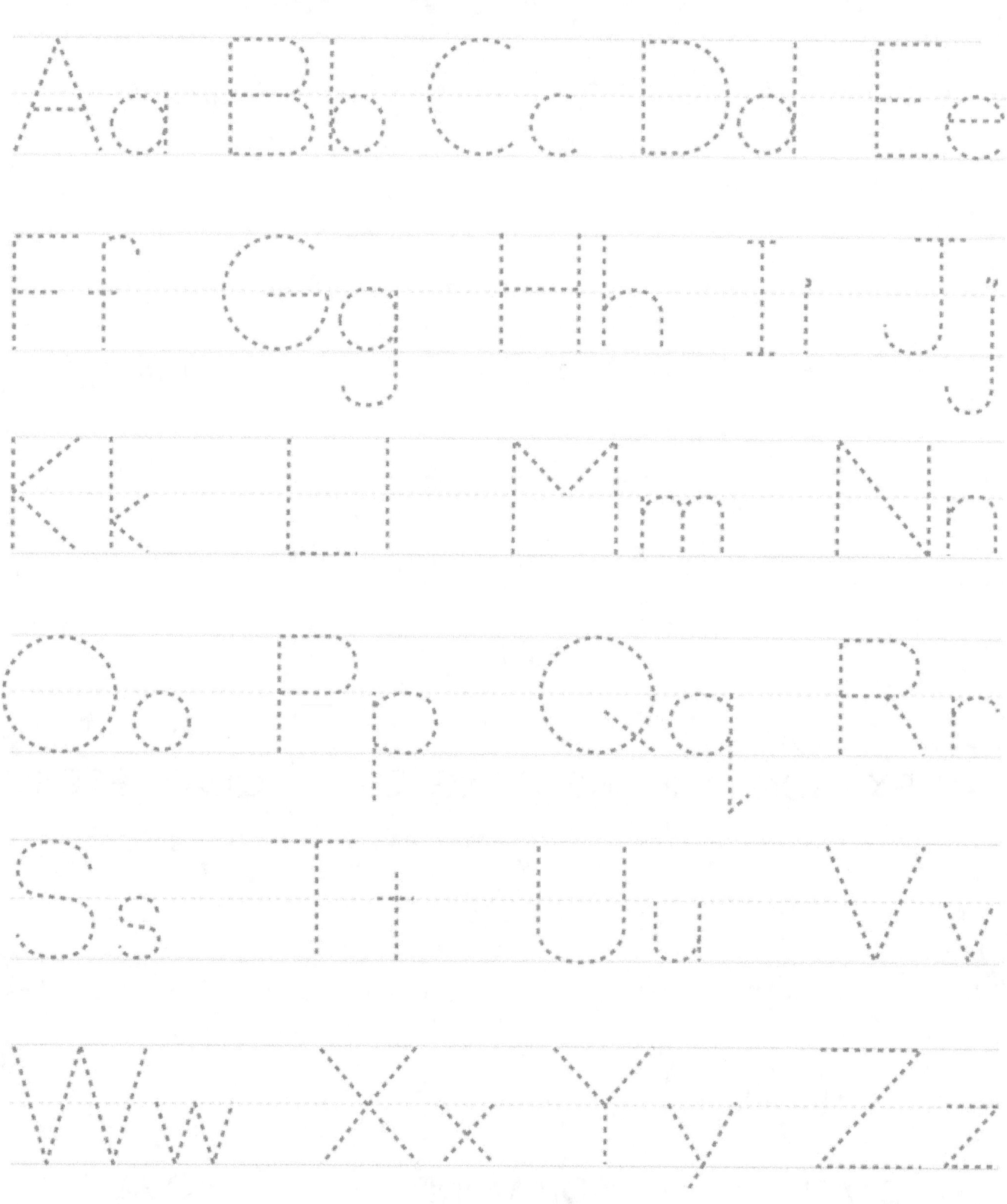

Trace the letters

Aa Bb Cc Dd Ee

Ff Gg Hh Ii Jj

Kk Ll Mm Nn

Oo Pp Qq Rr

Ss Tt Uu Vv

Ww Xx Yy Zz

Trace the letters

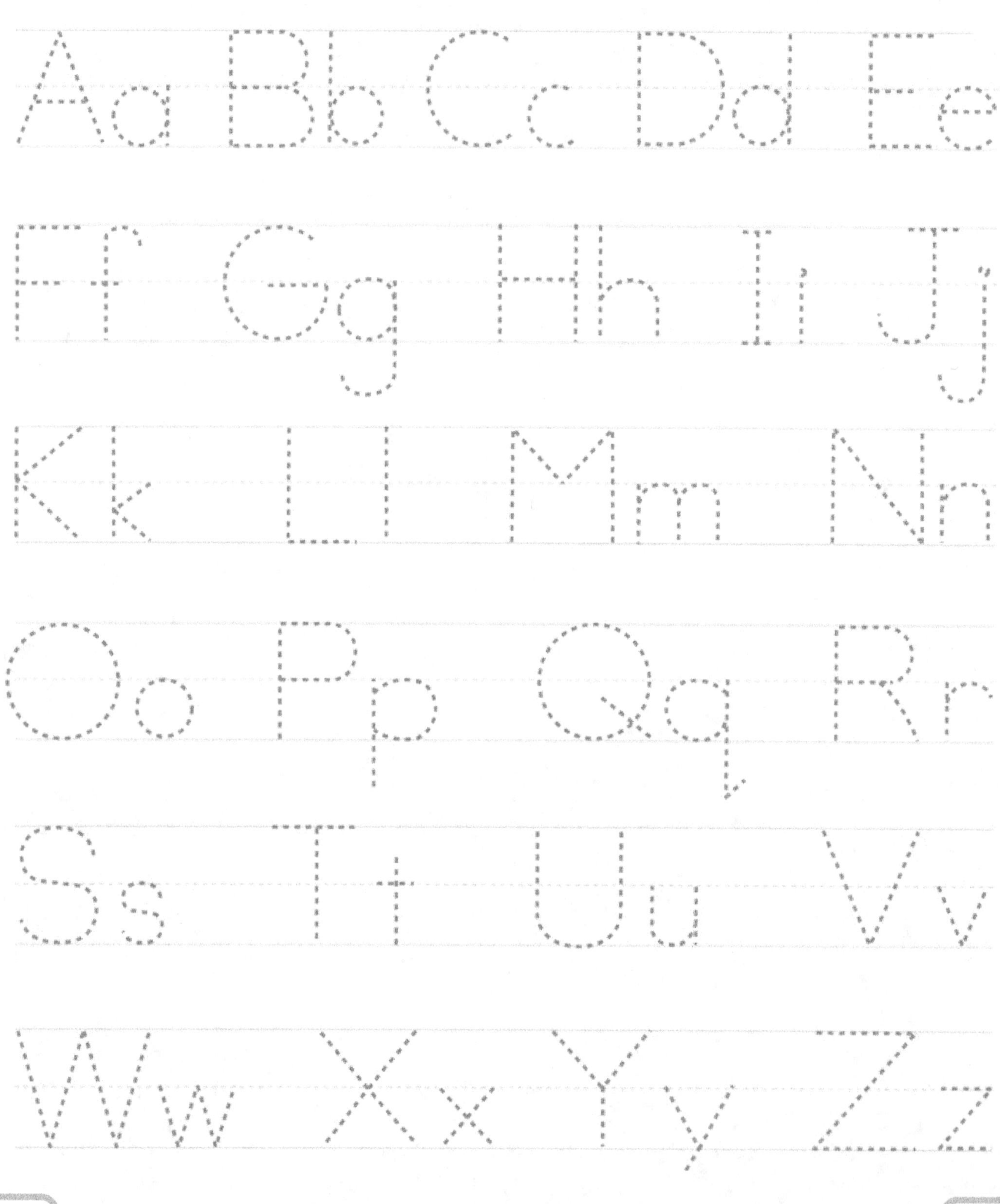

Trace the numbers

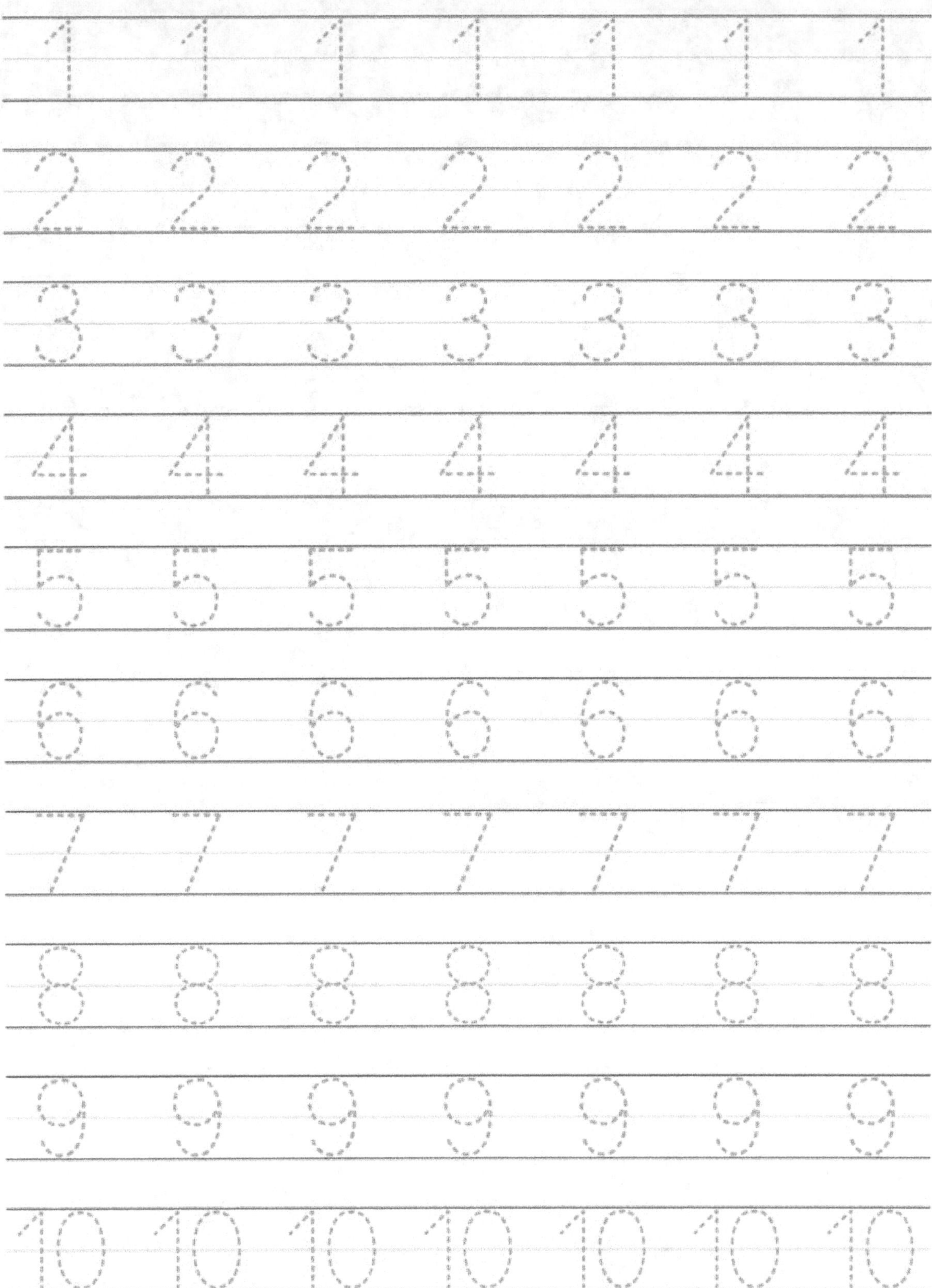

Trace the numbers

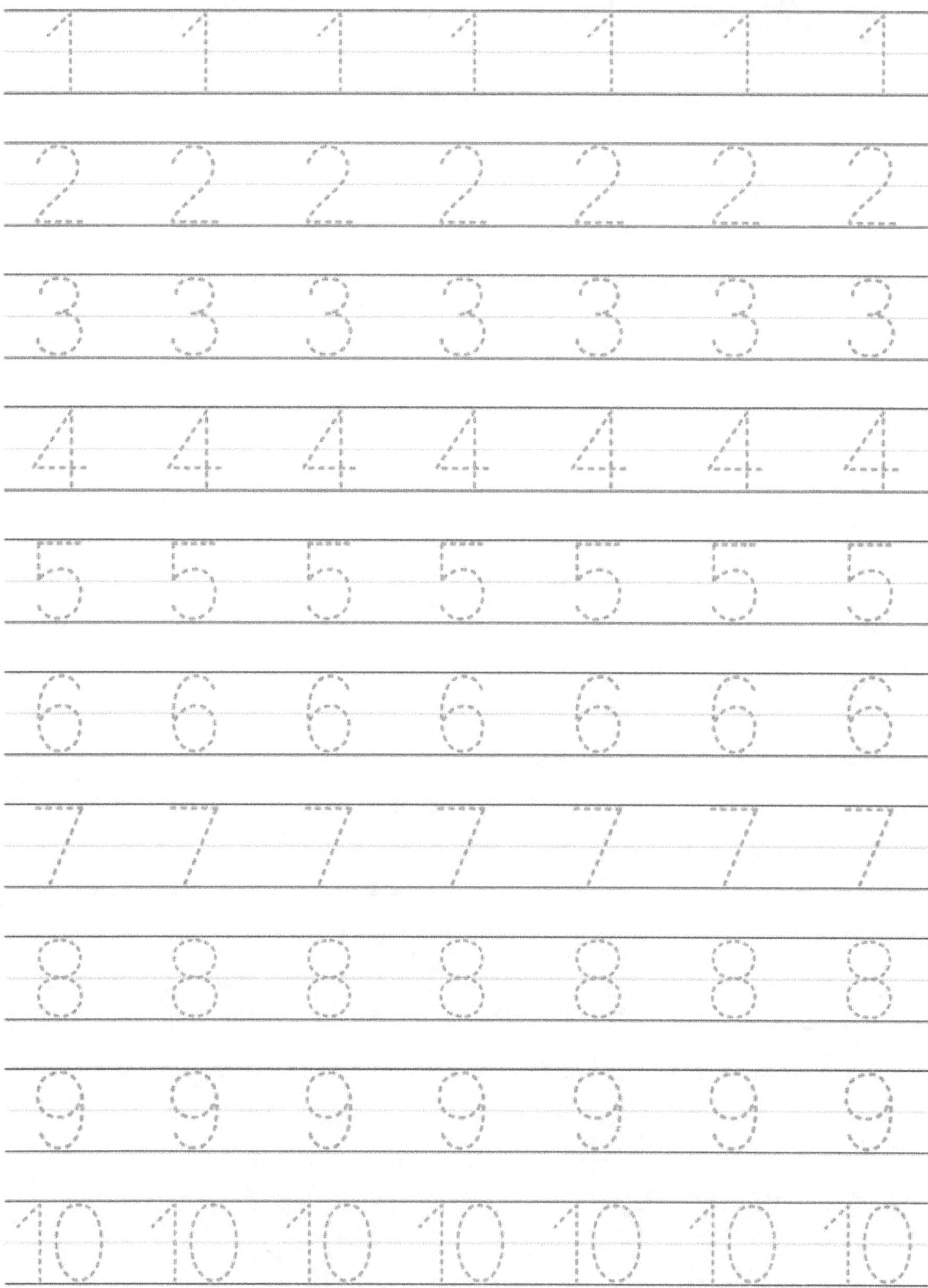

Trace the numbers

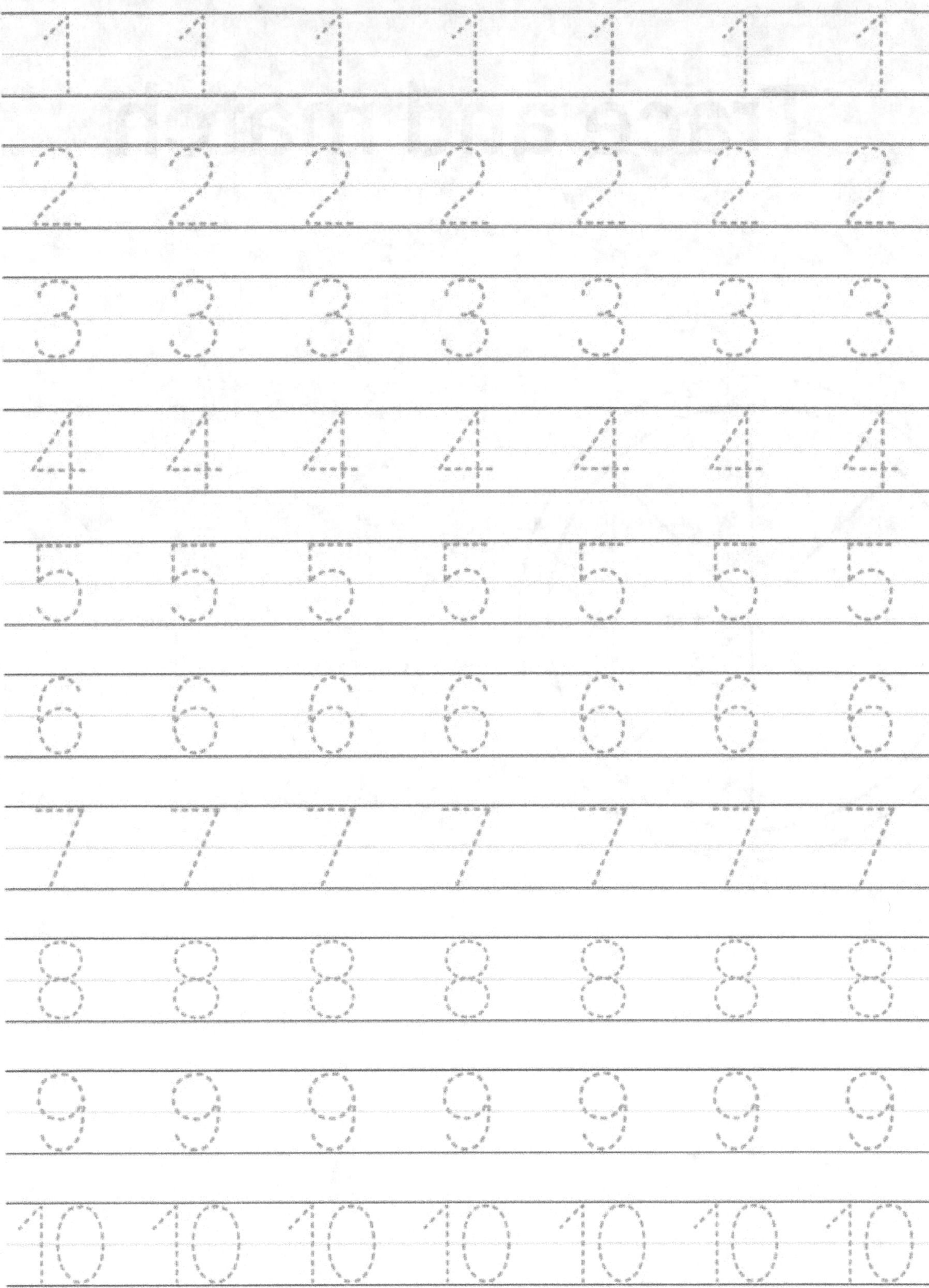

Trace and match

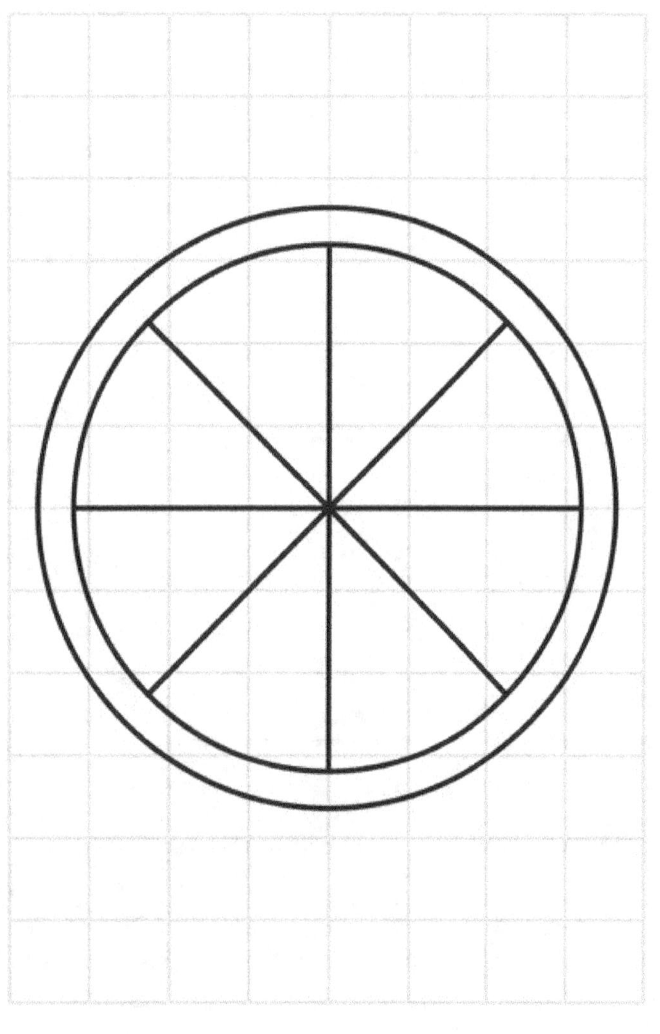 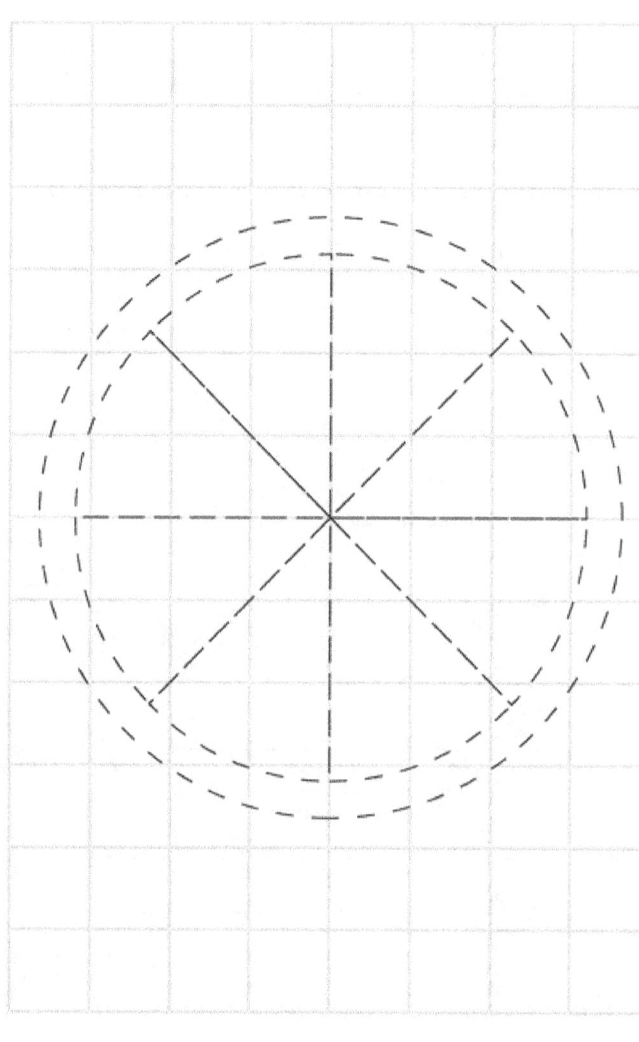

Trace and match

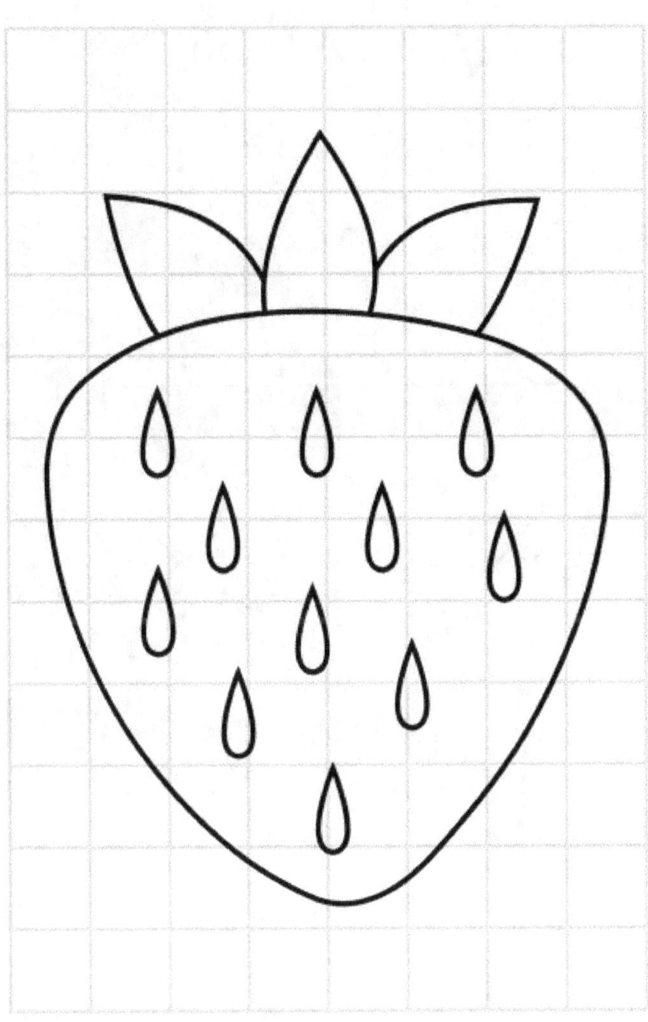 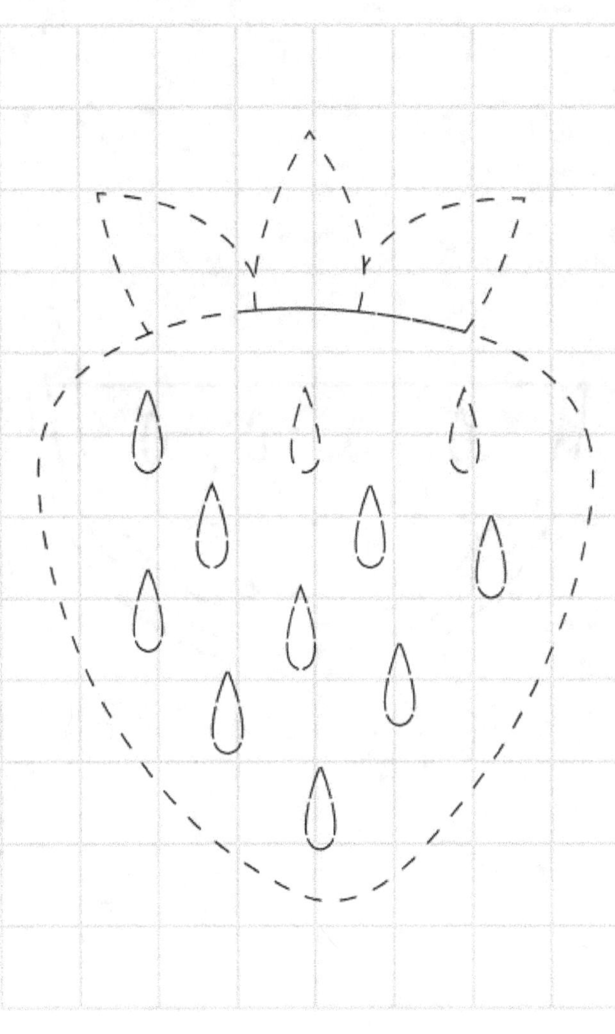

Trace and match

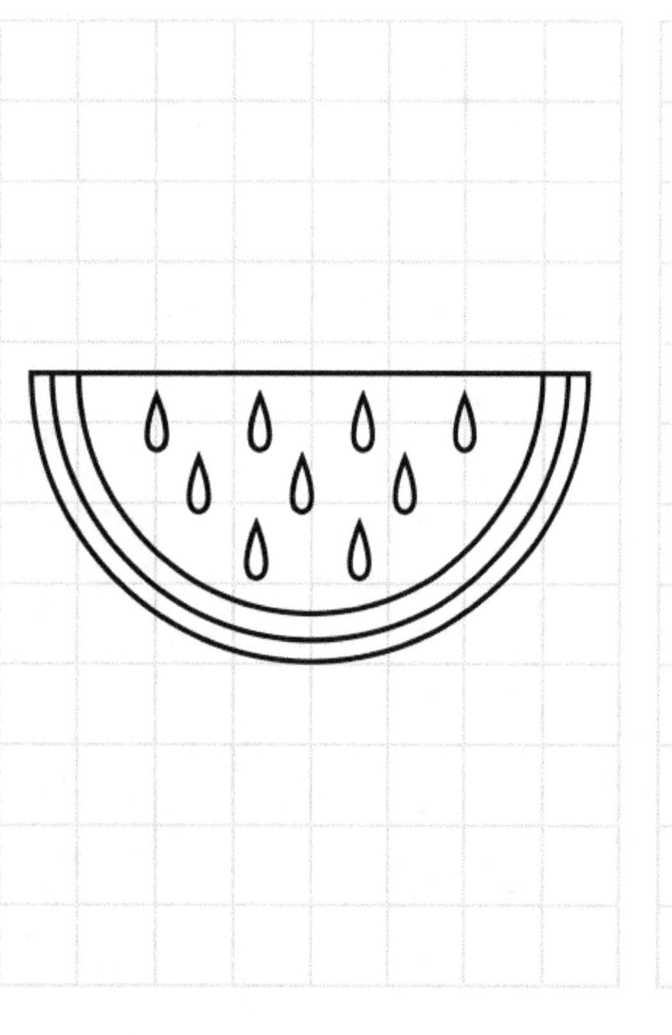 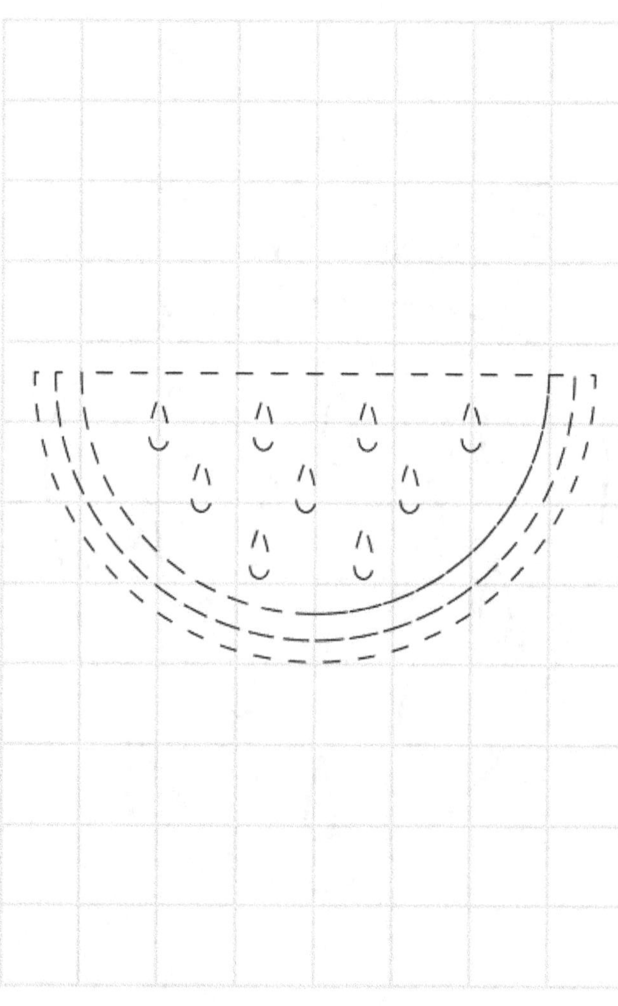

Connect the dots

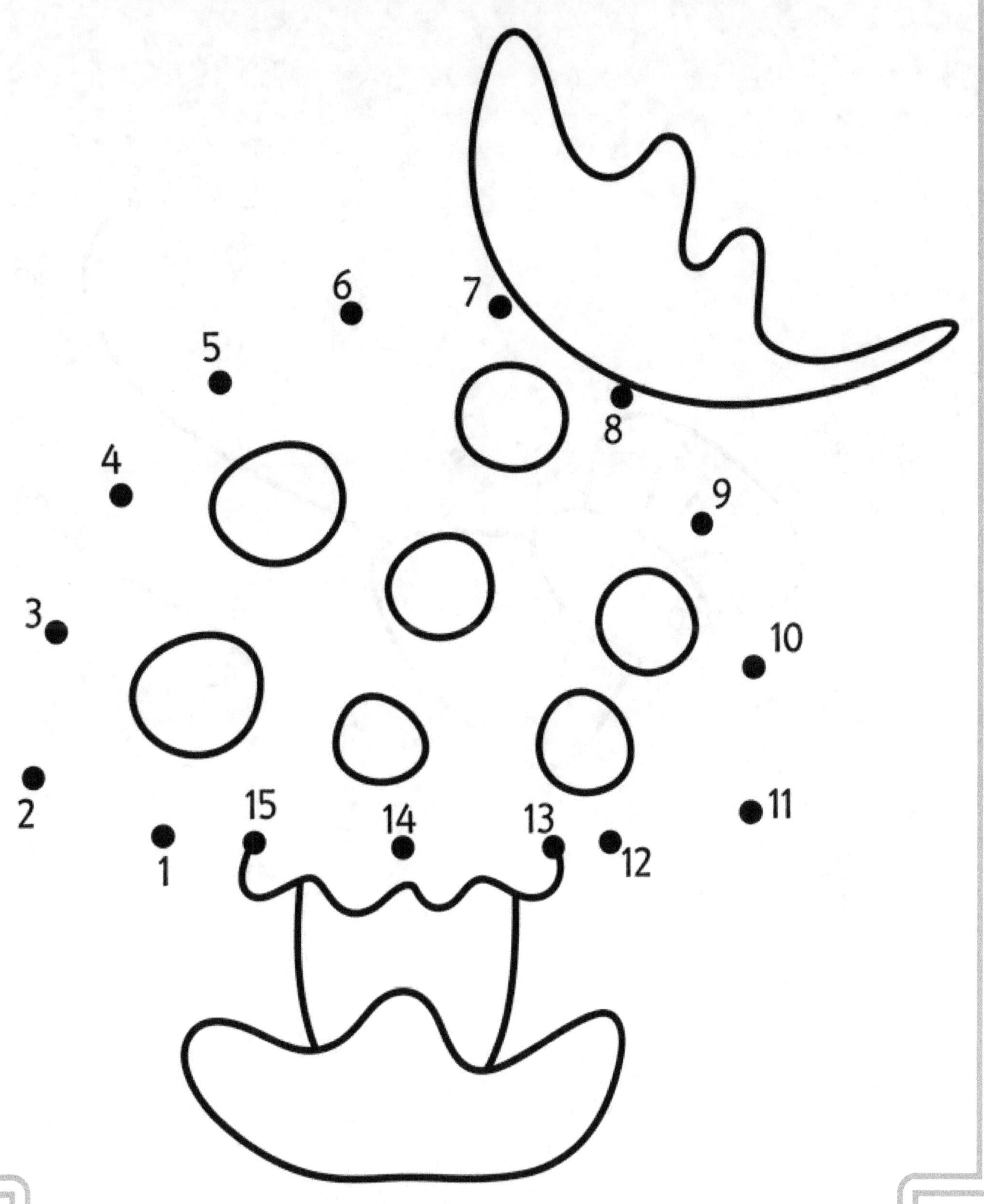

Connect the dots

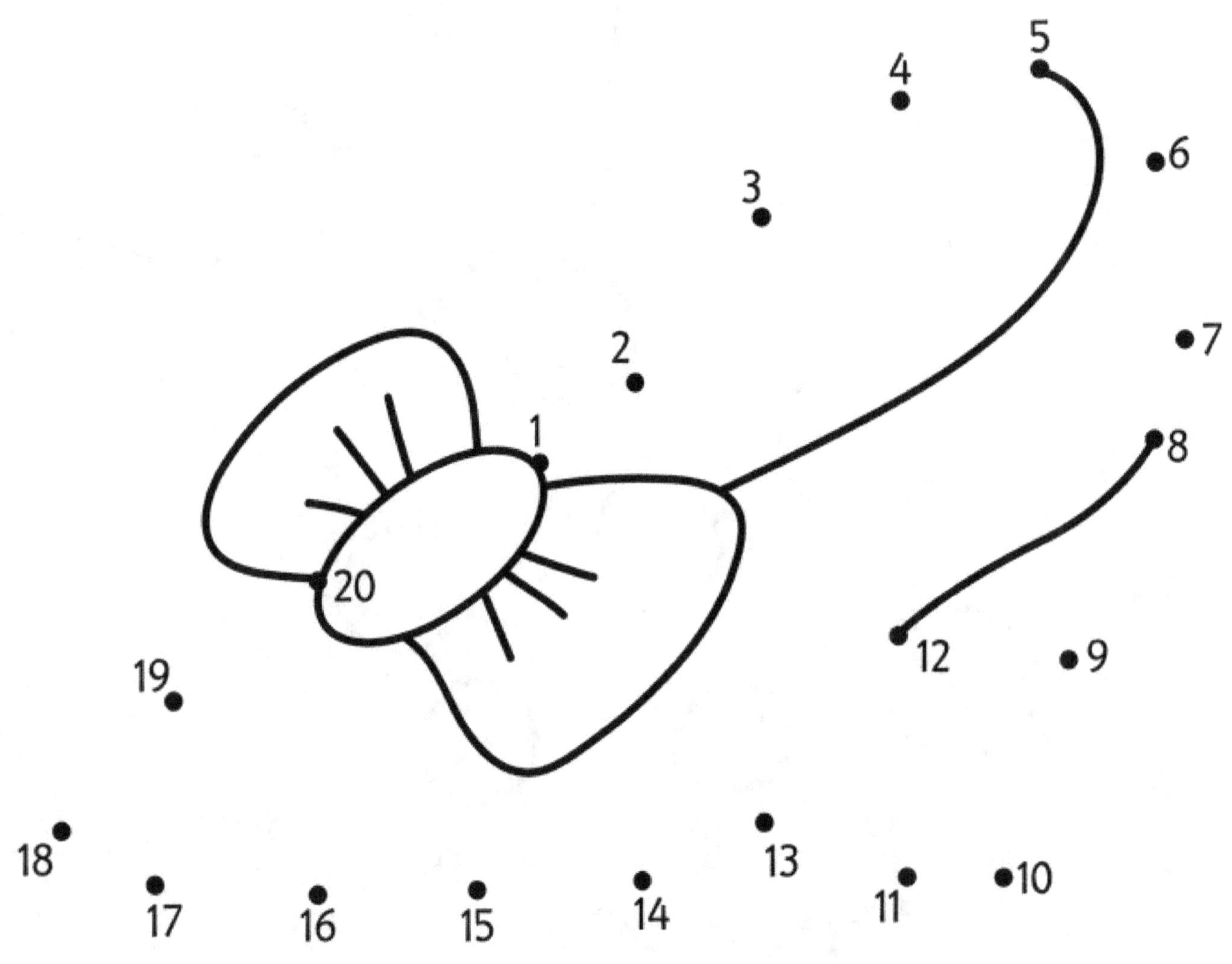

Connect the dots

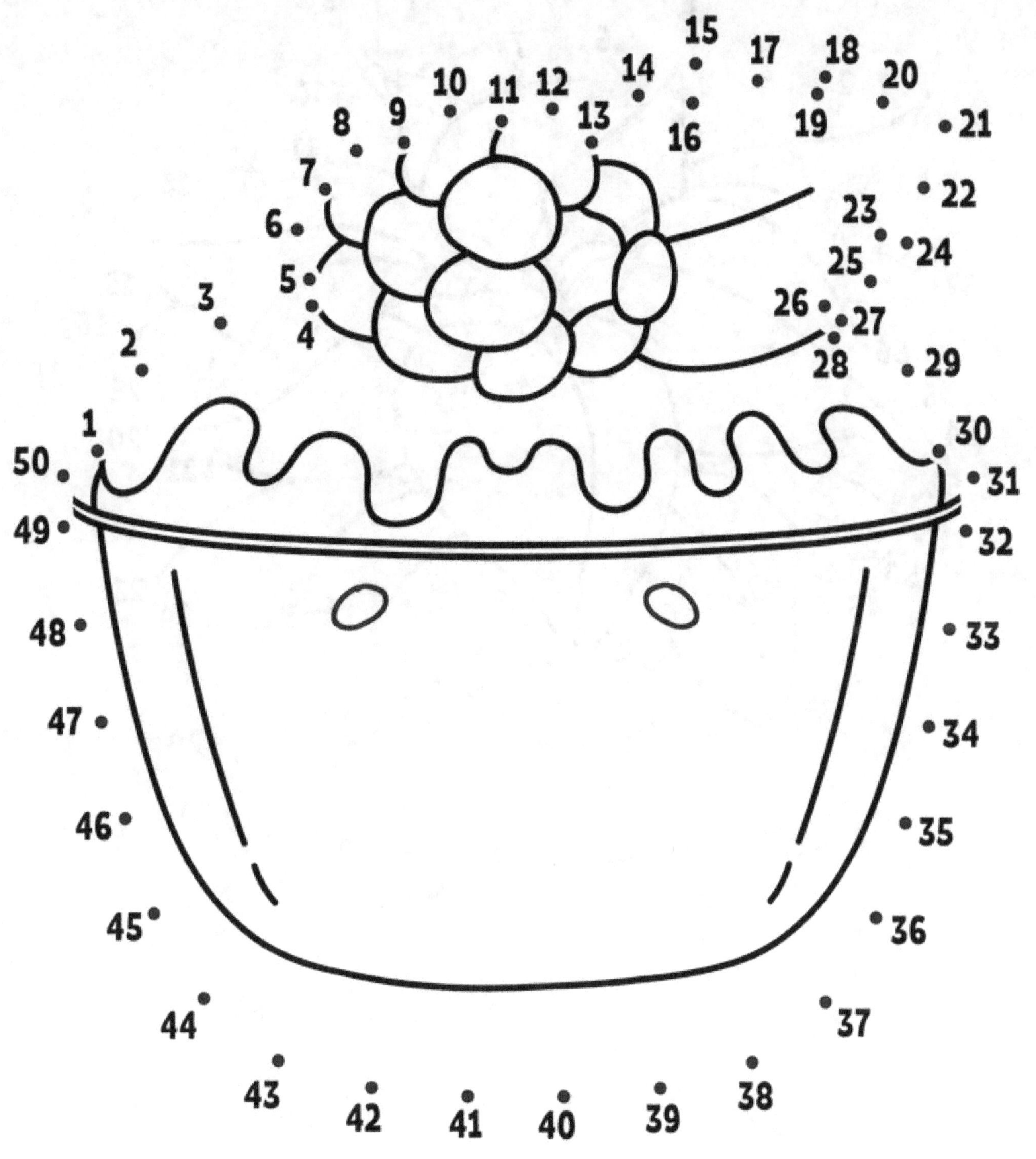

Connect the dots

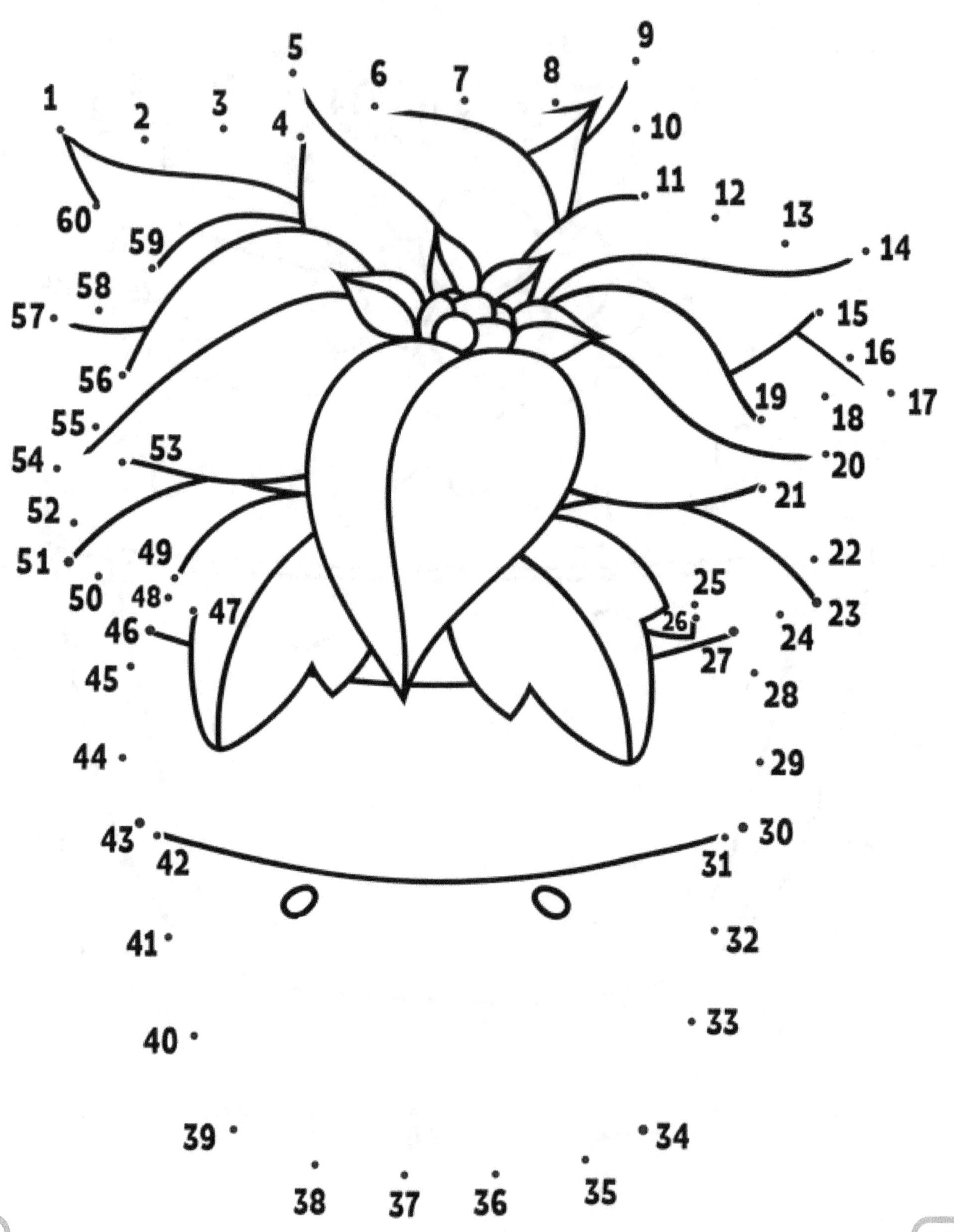

Symmetry drawing

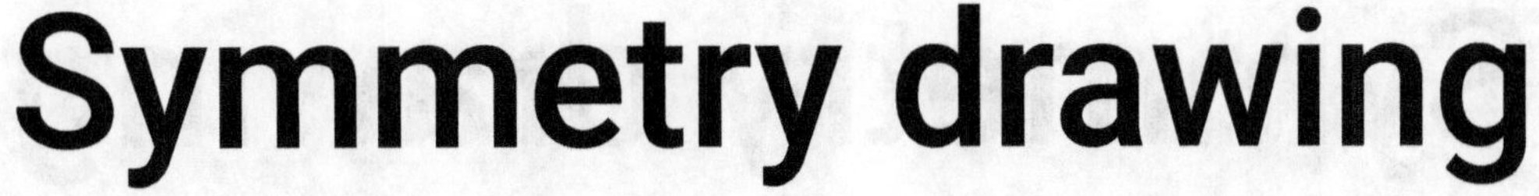

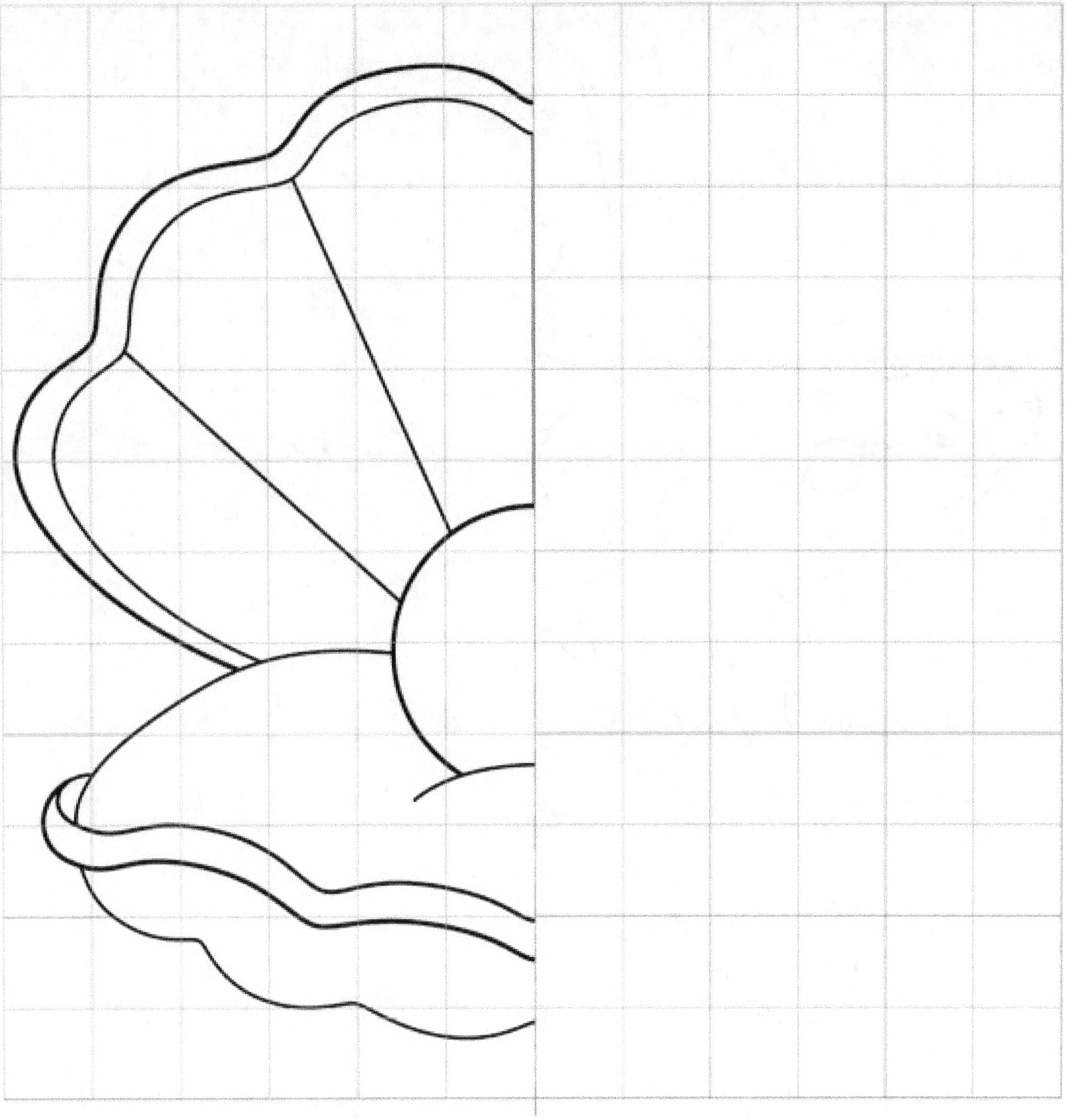

Symmetry drawing

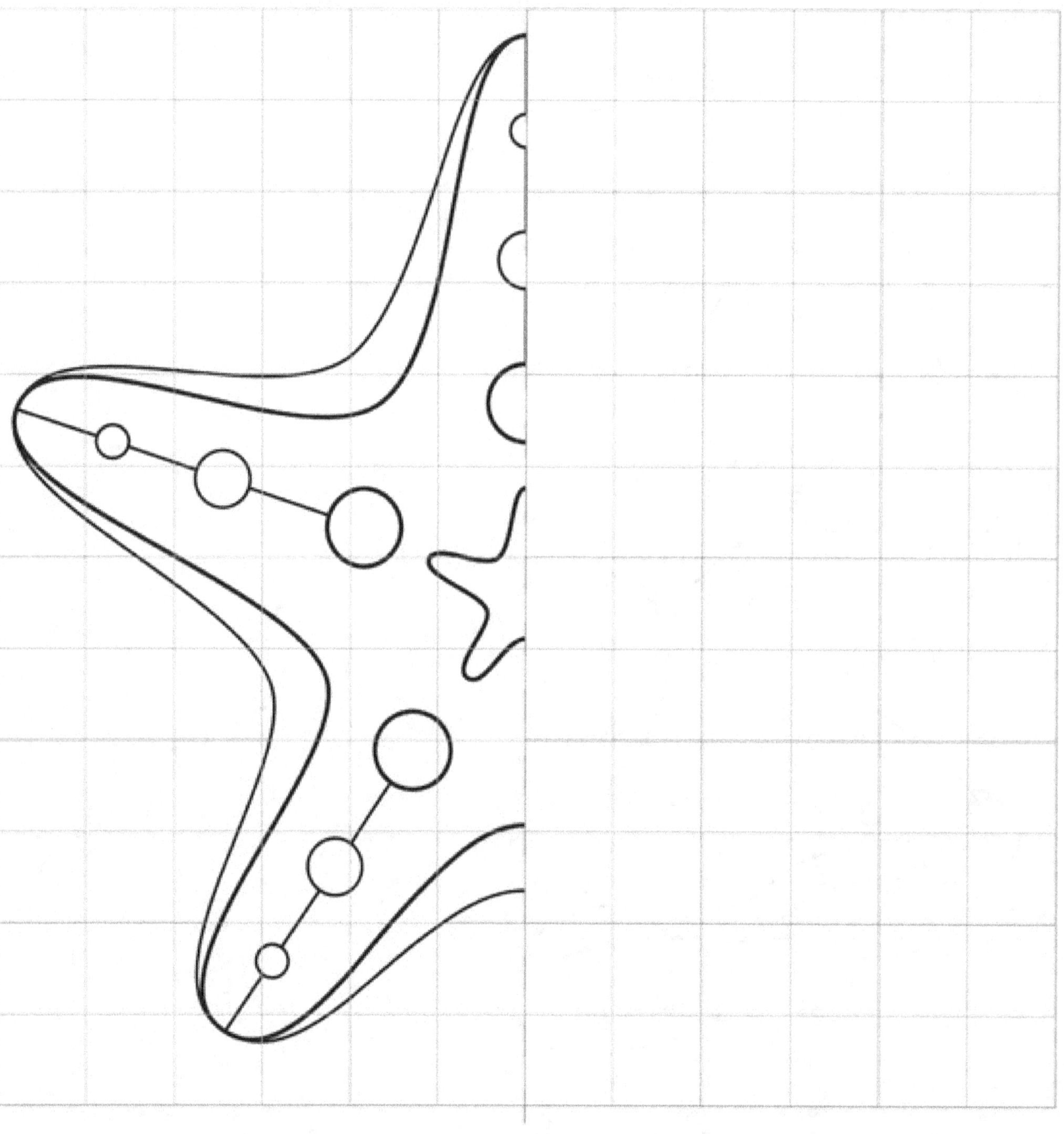

Symmetry drawing

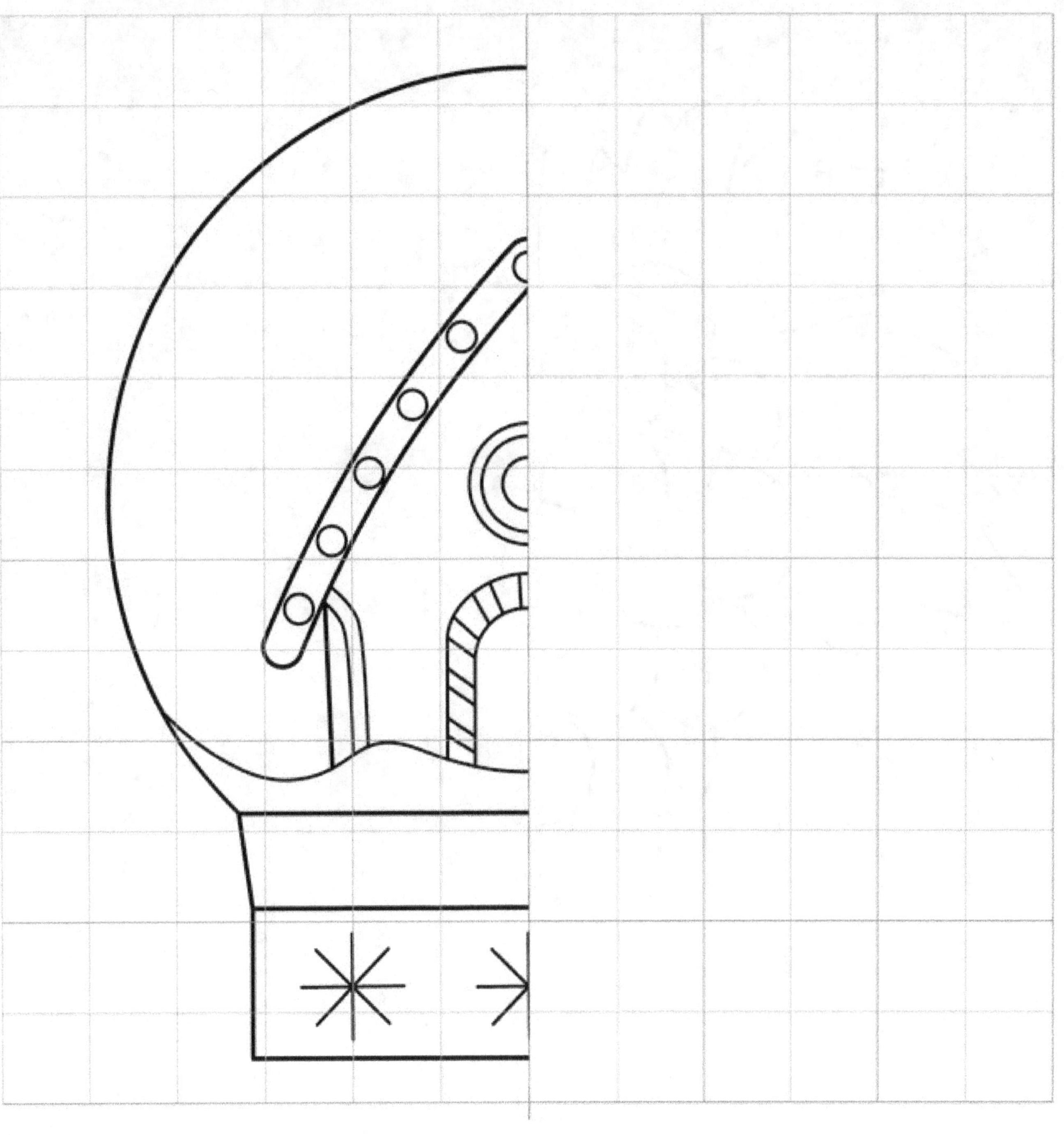

Symmetry drawing

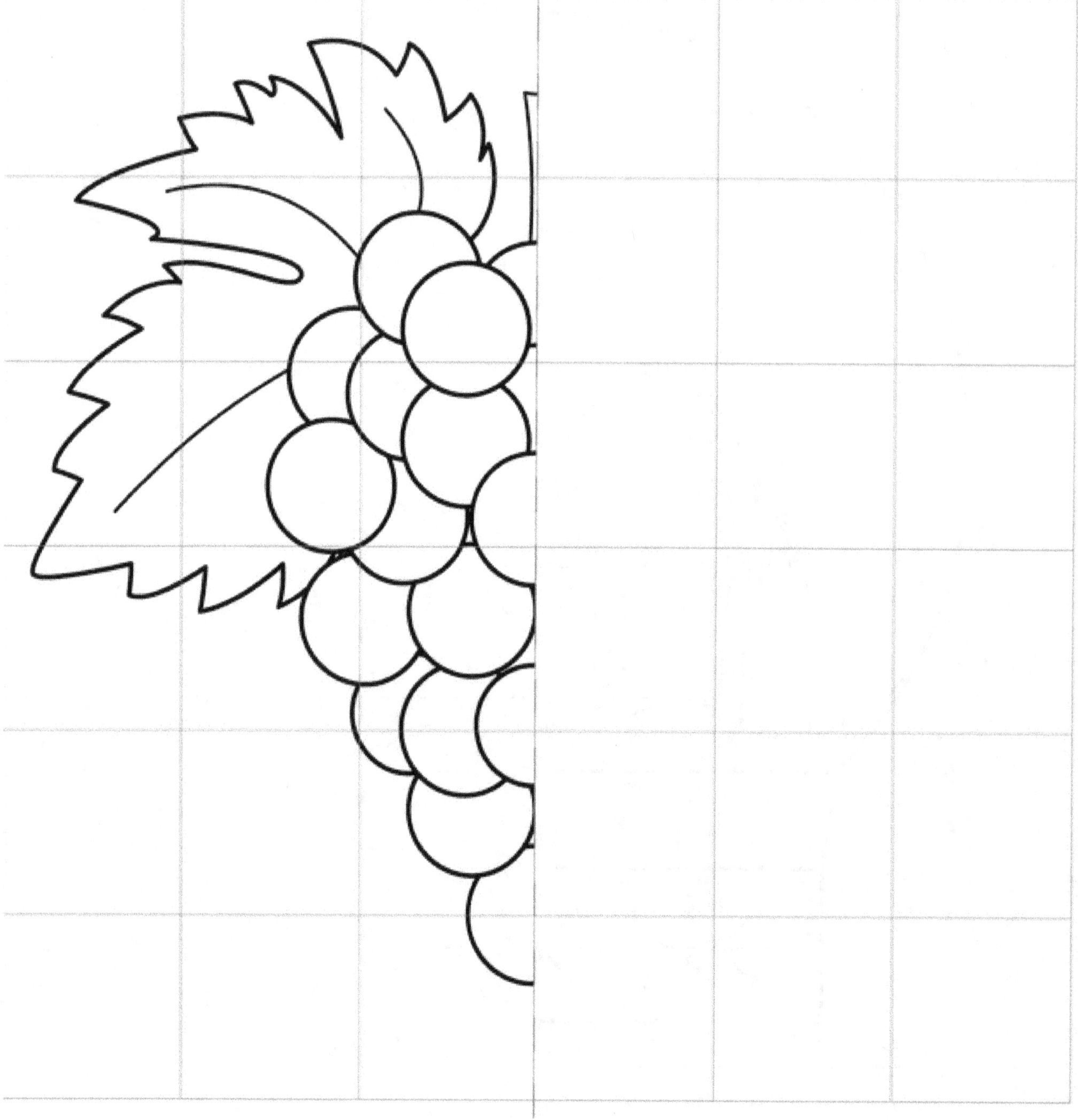

Shadow matching

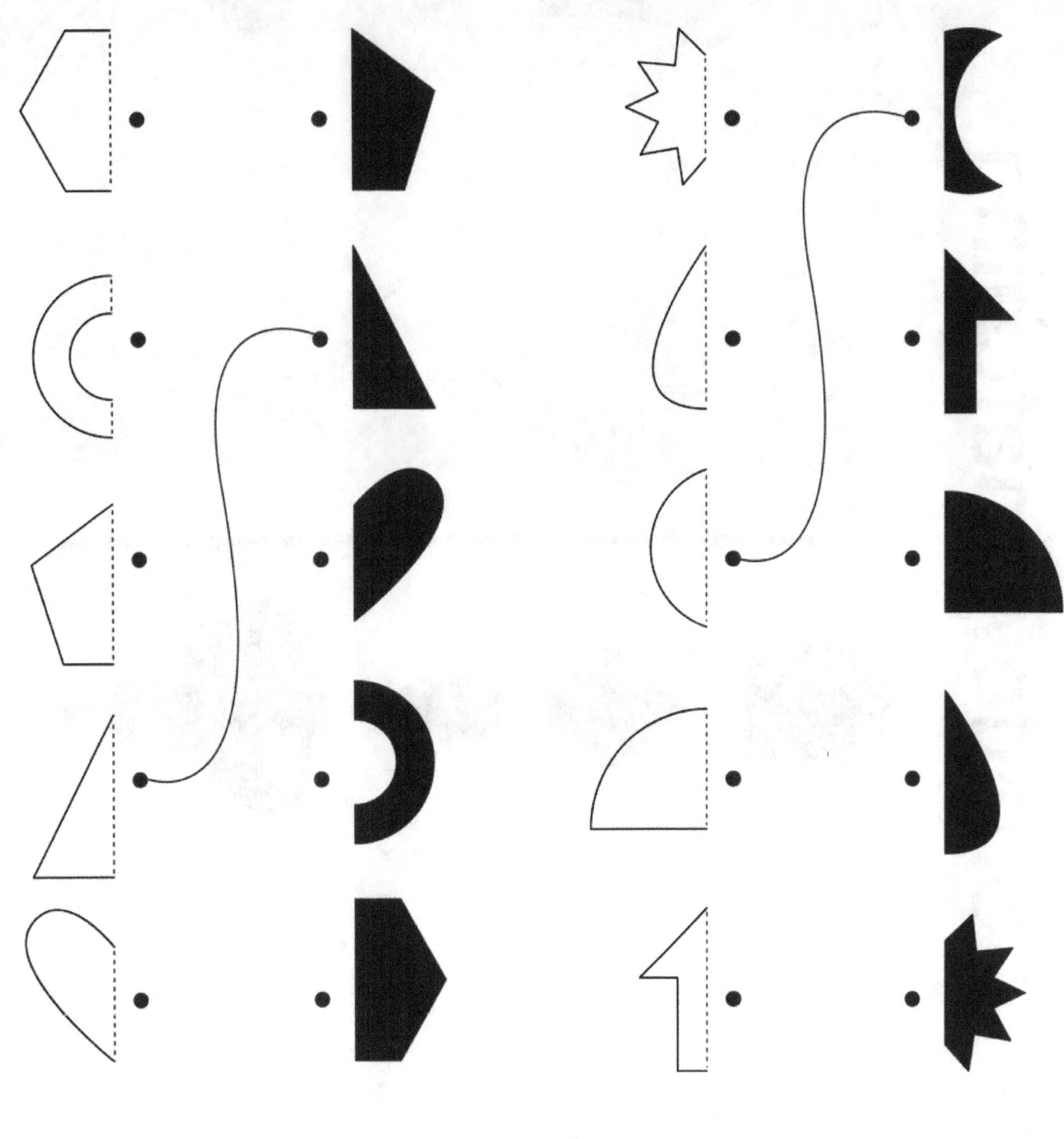

Shadow matching

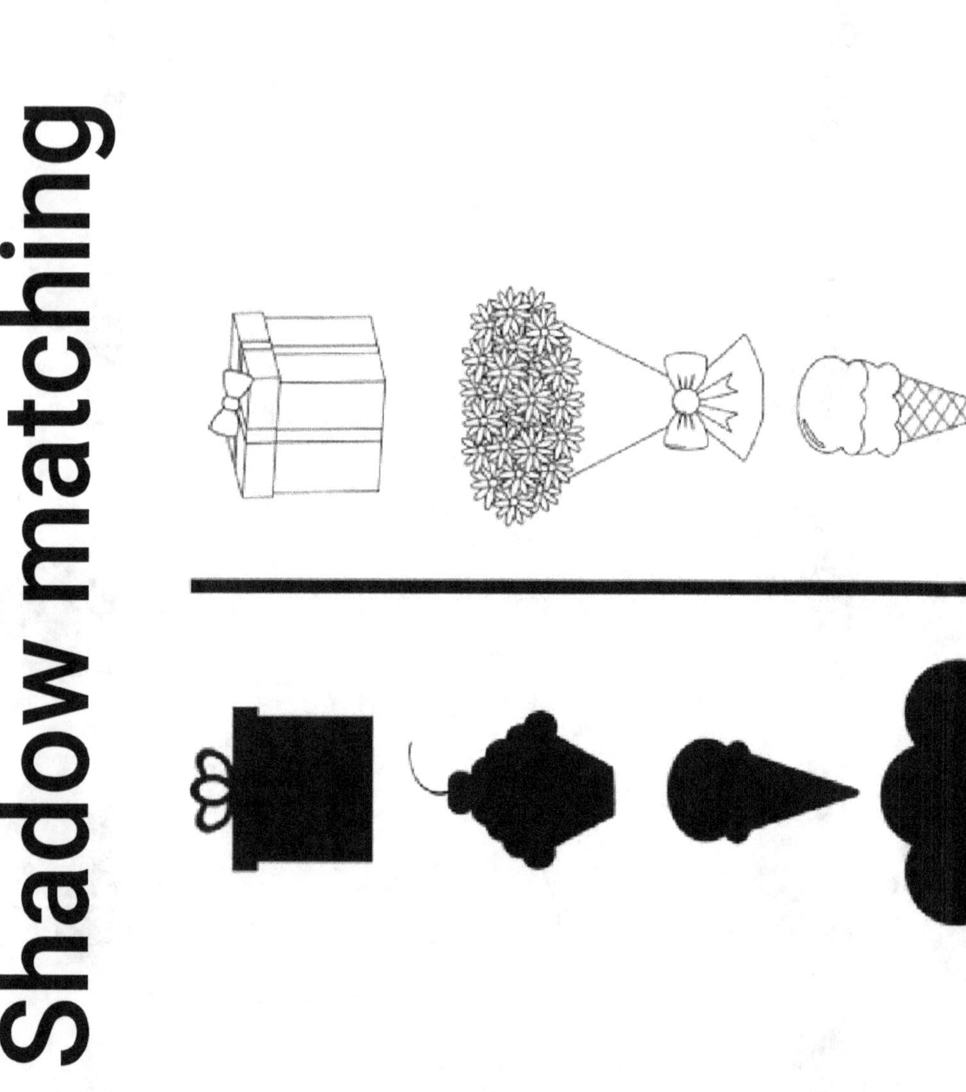

Shadow matching

Shadow matching

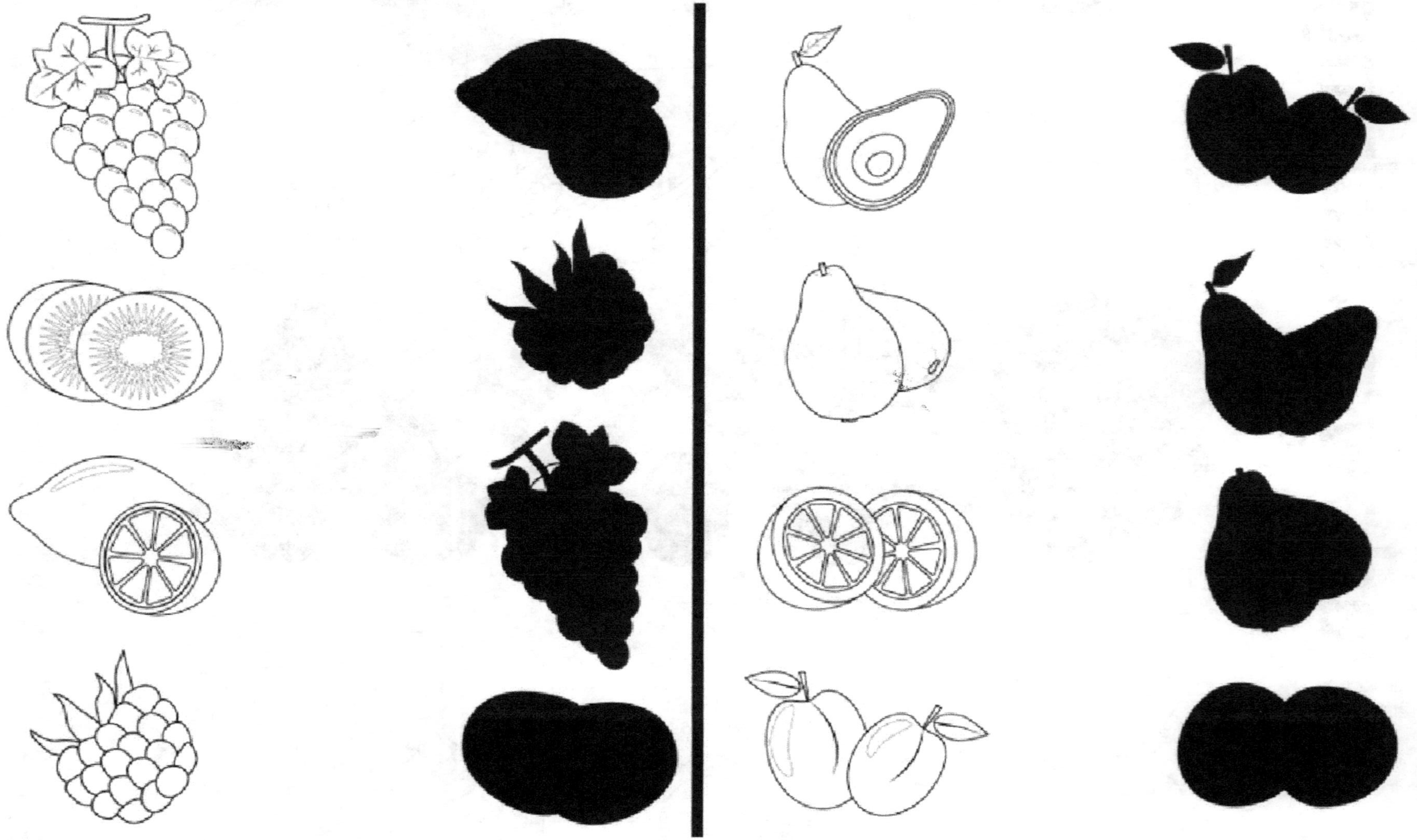

Item hunt

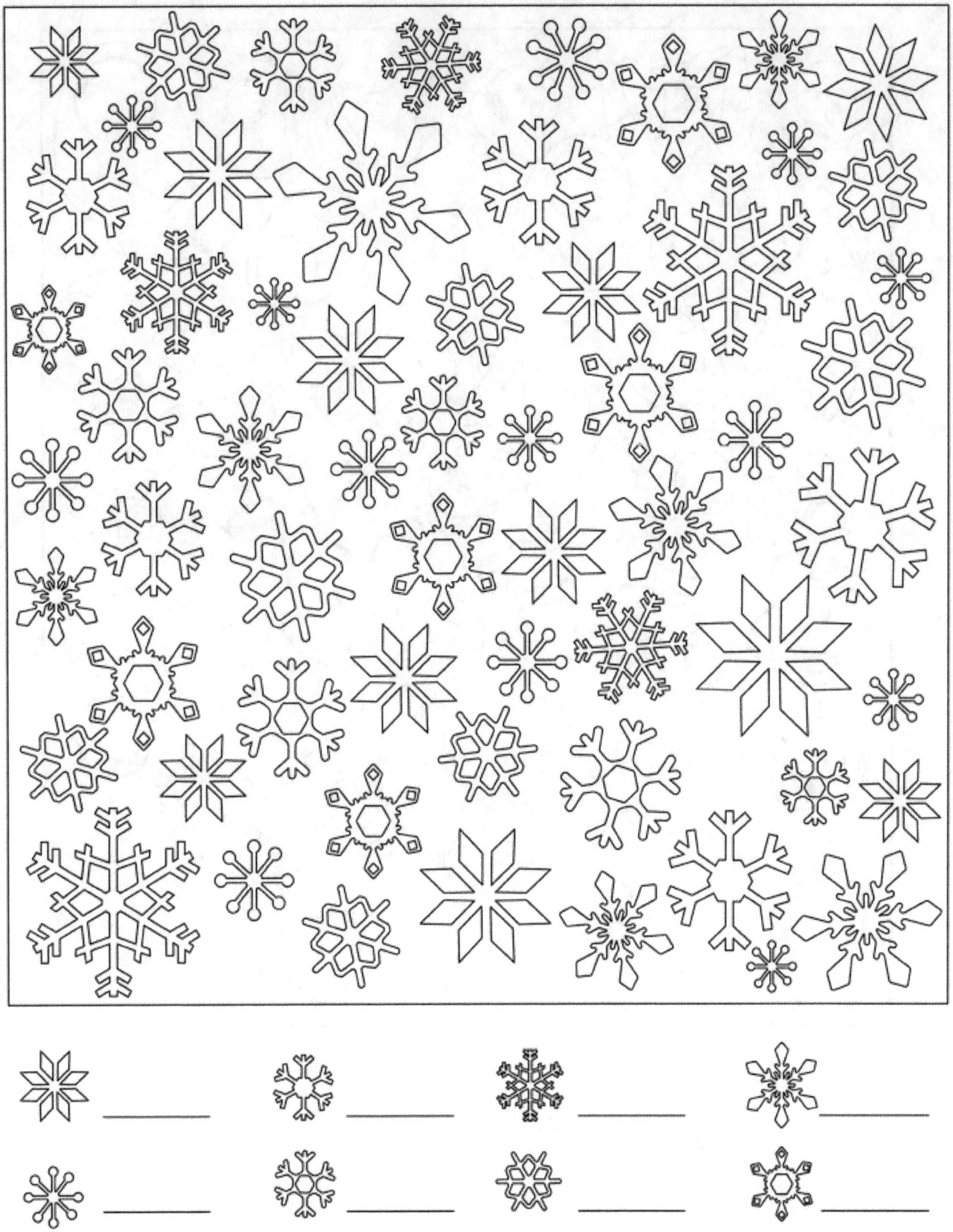

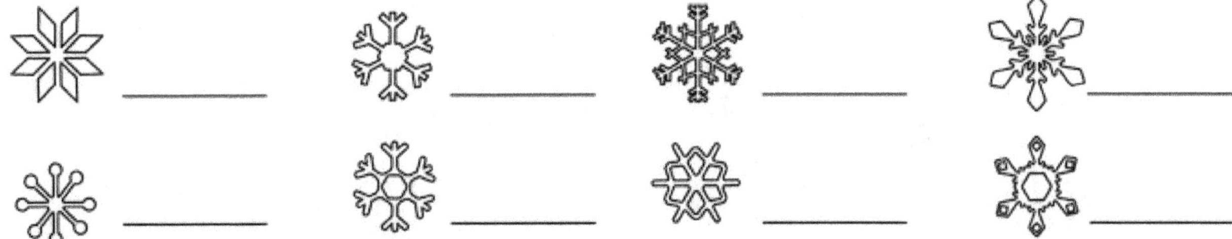

Item hunt

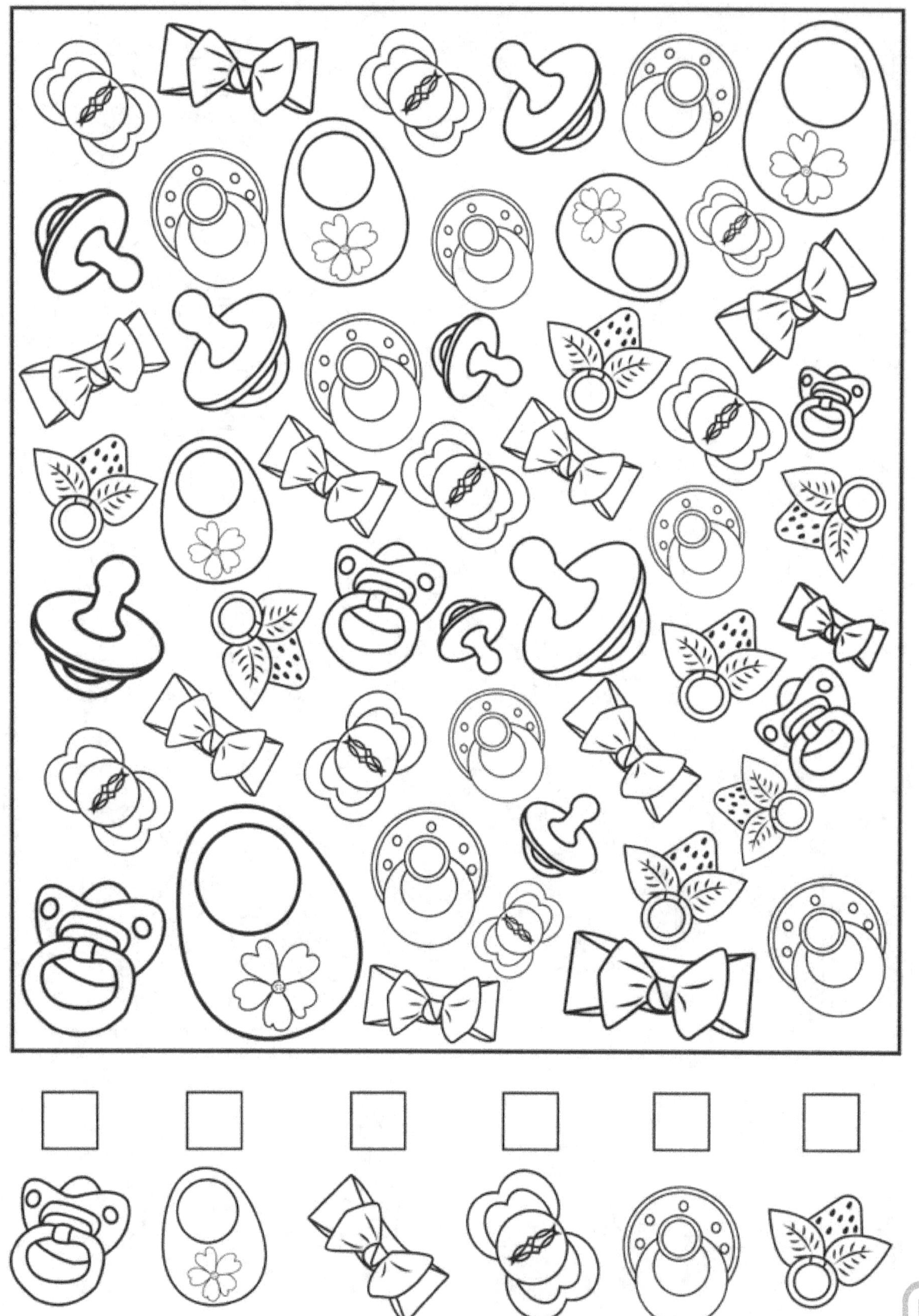

Item hunt

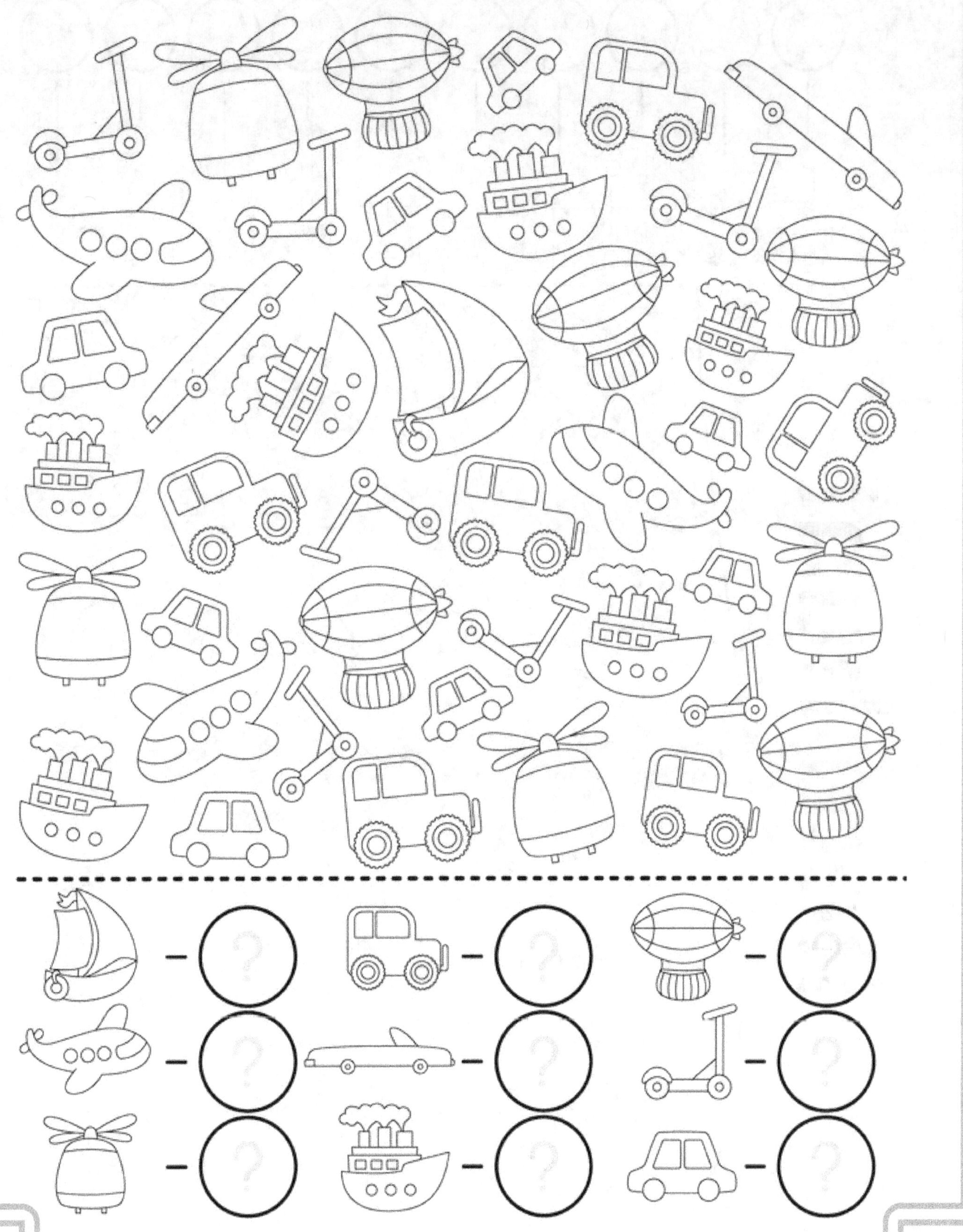

Item hunt

Item hunt

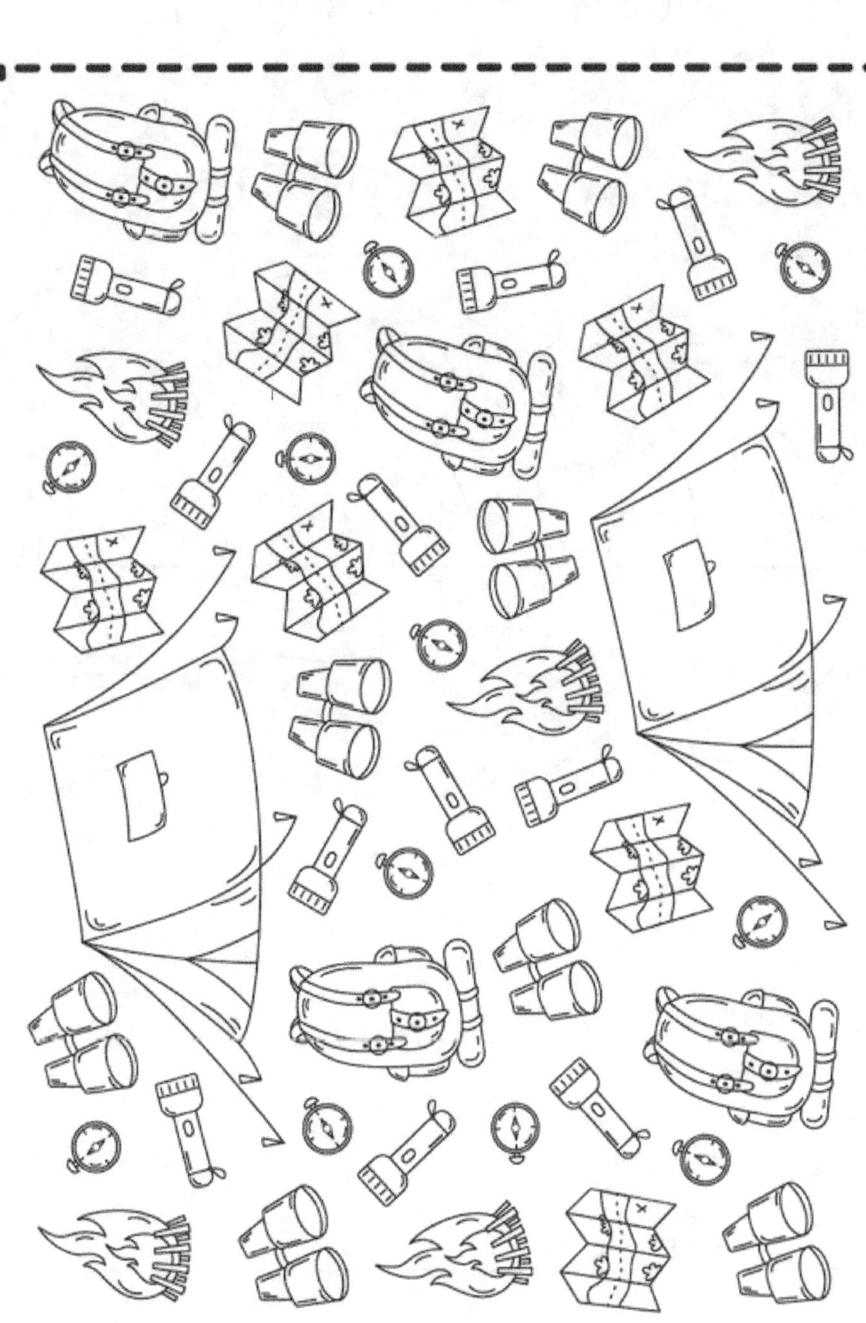

Coloring pages

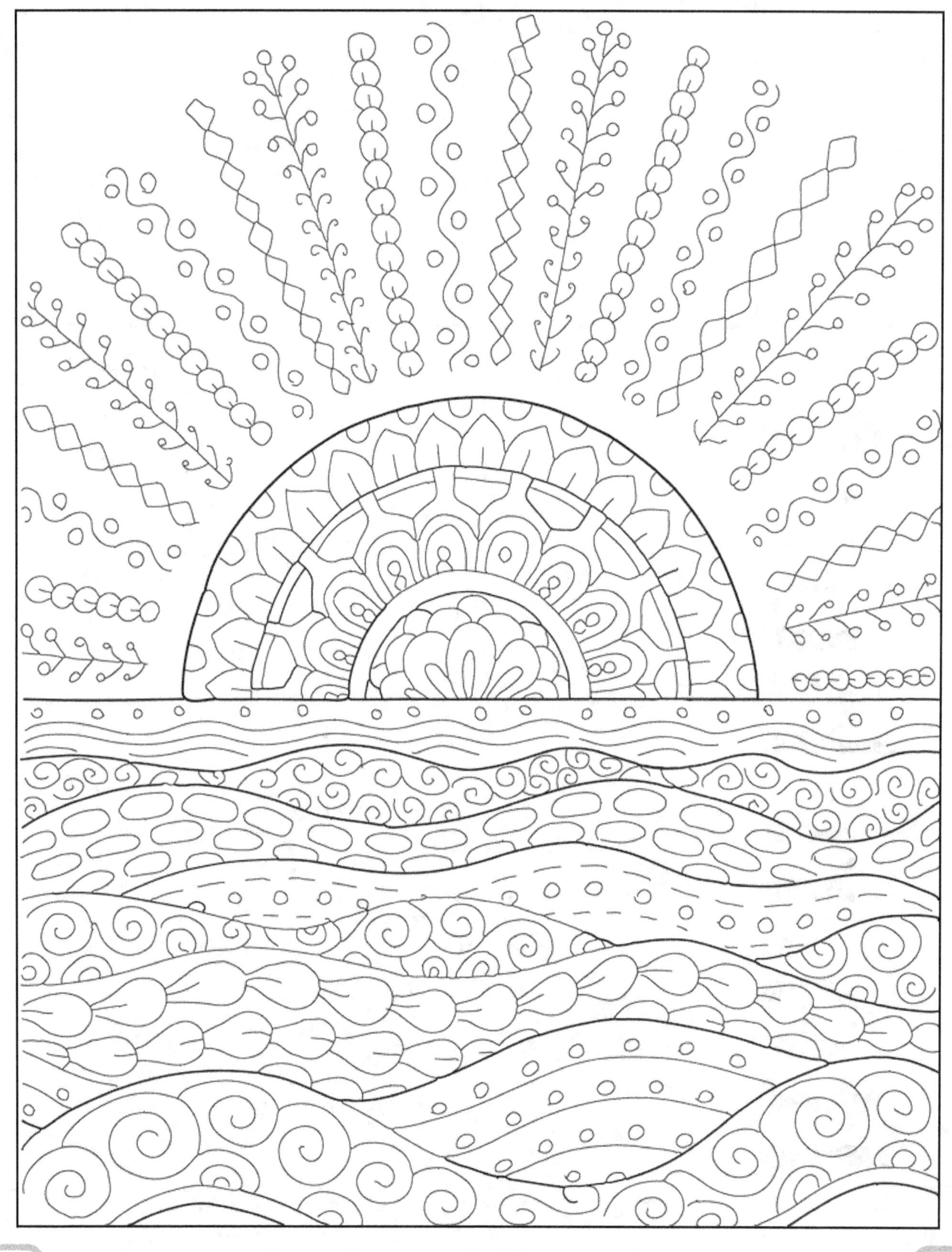

Coloring pages

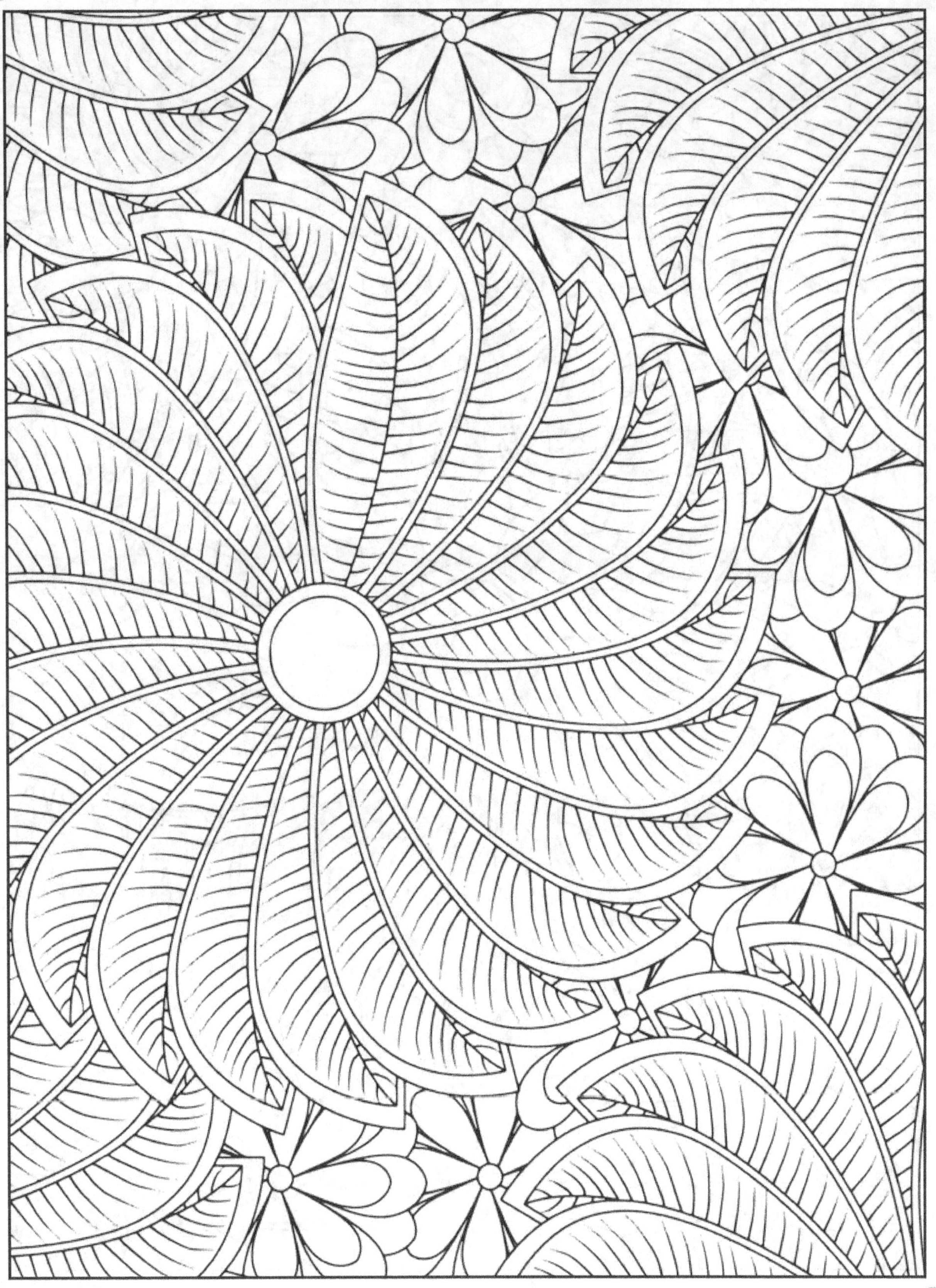

Coloring pages

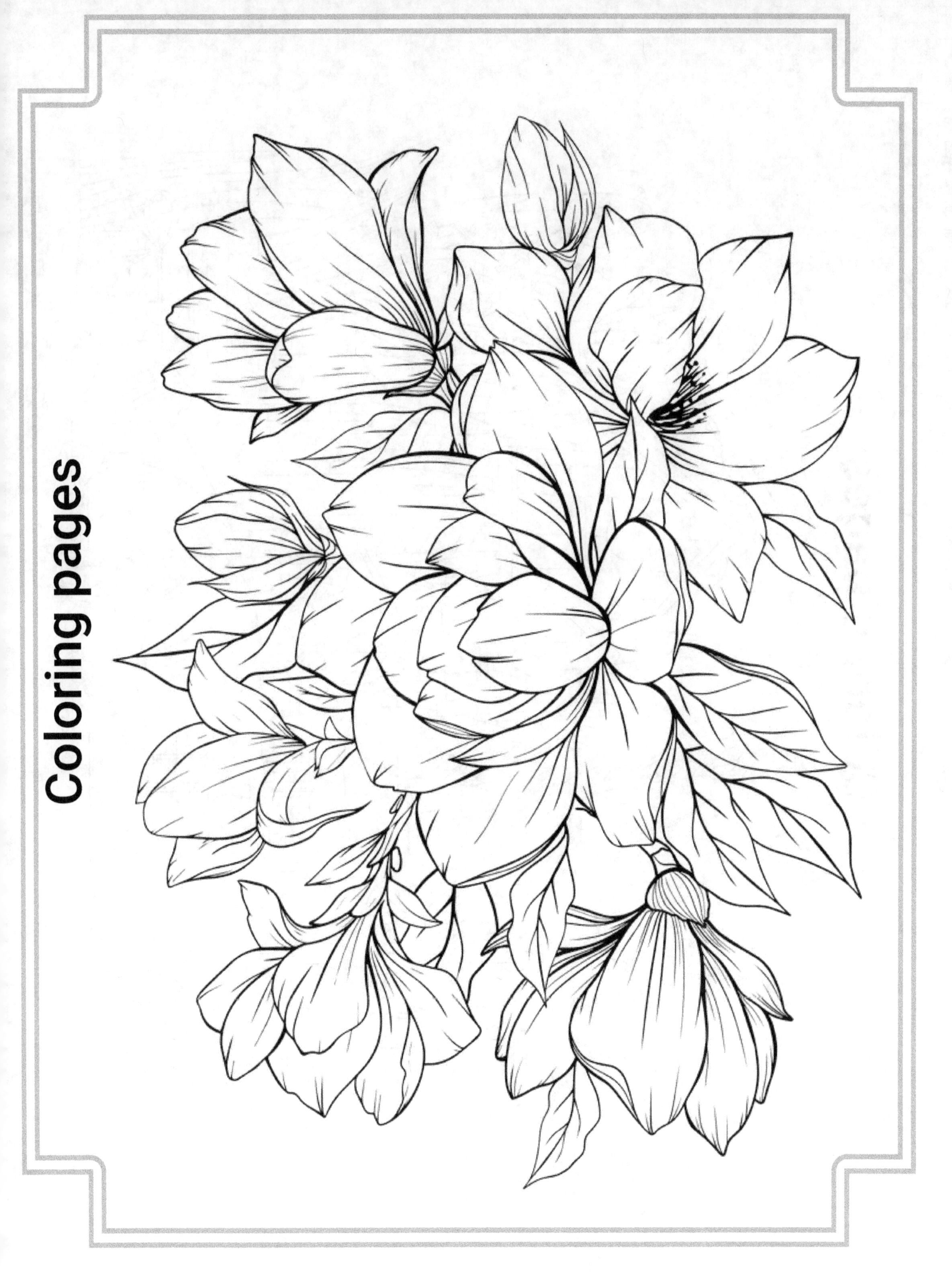
Coloring pages

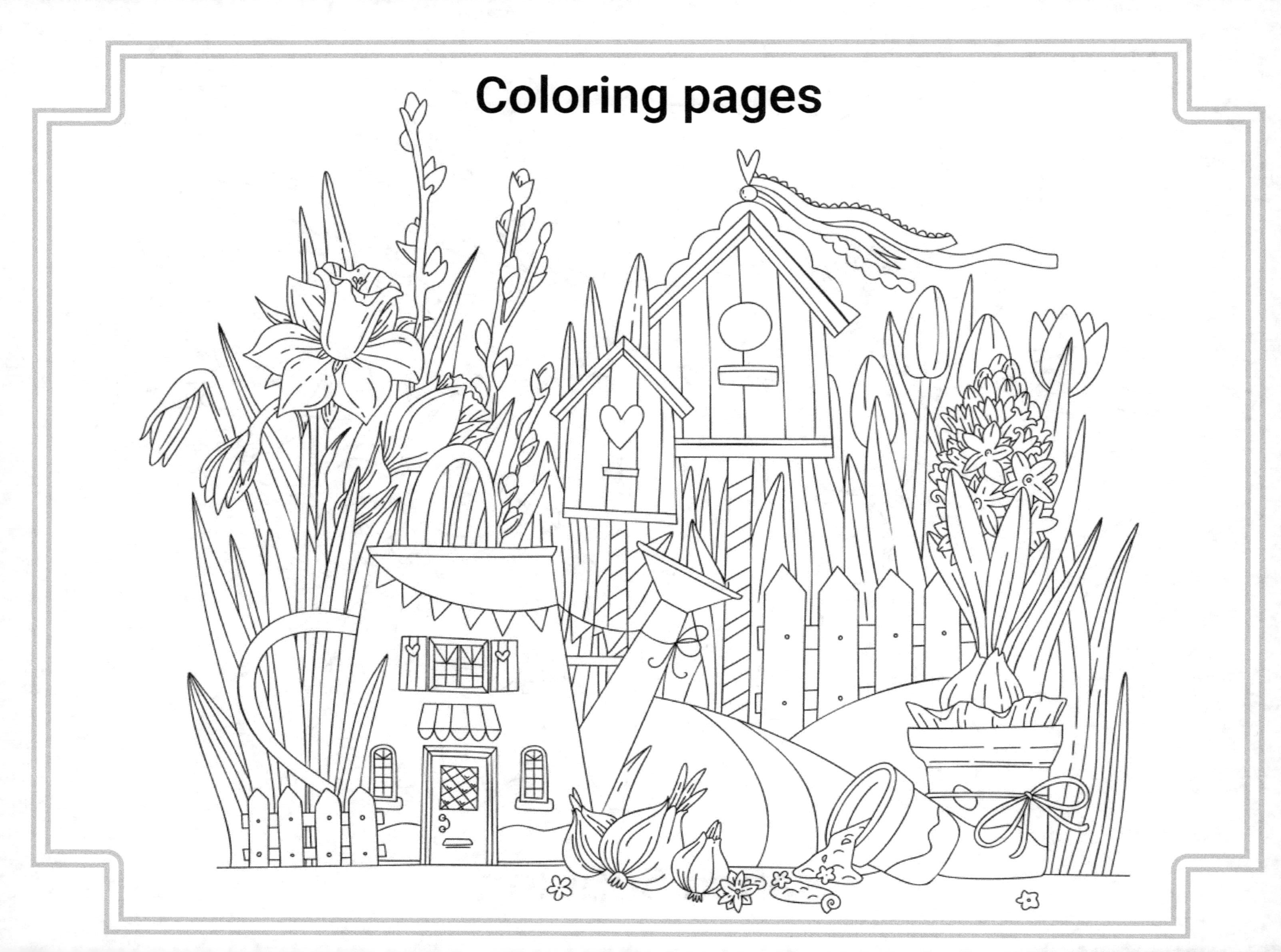

Coloring pages

Coloring pages

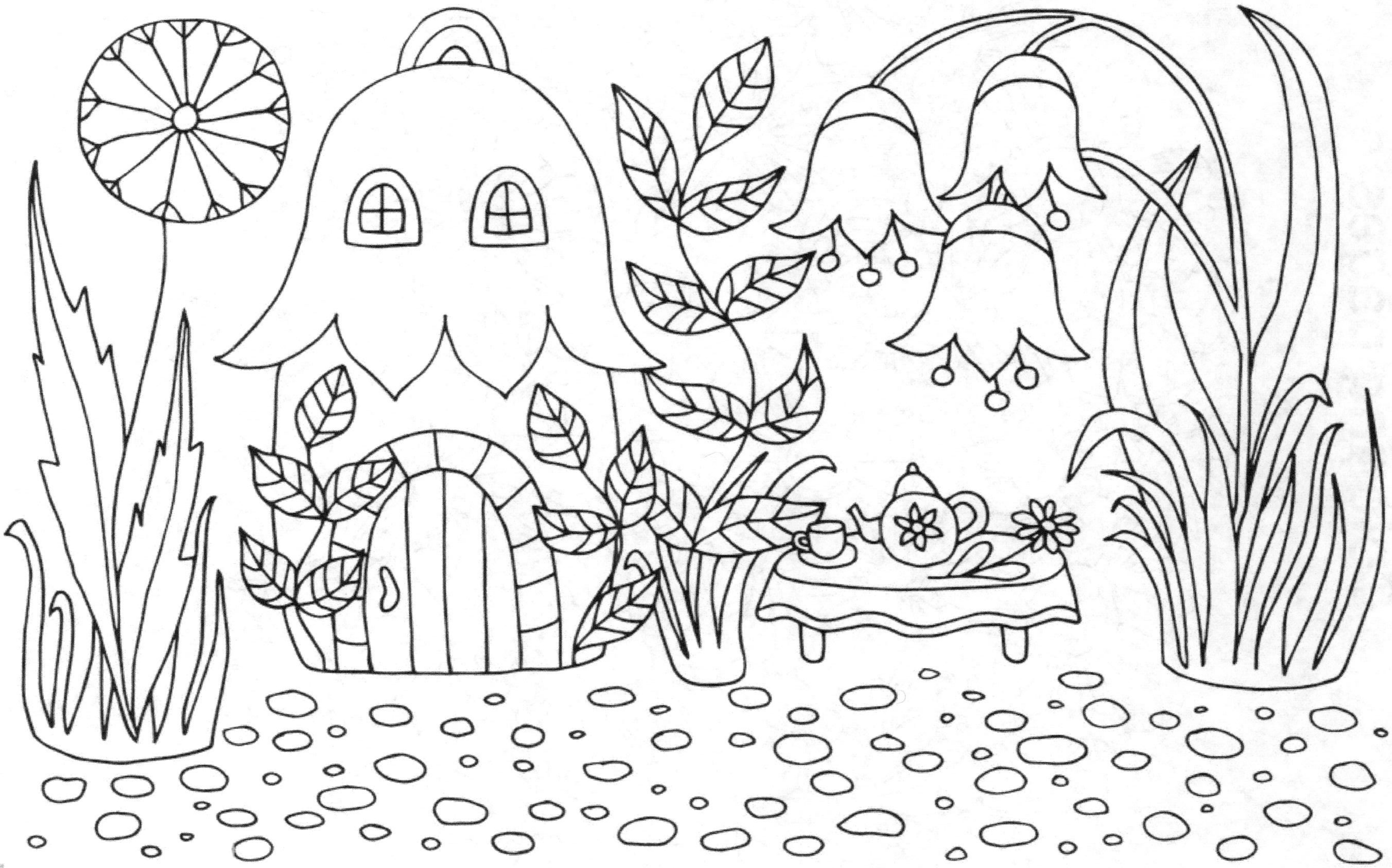

Coloring pages

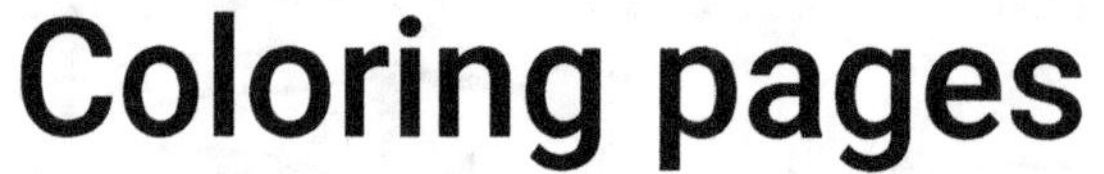

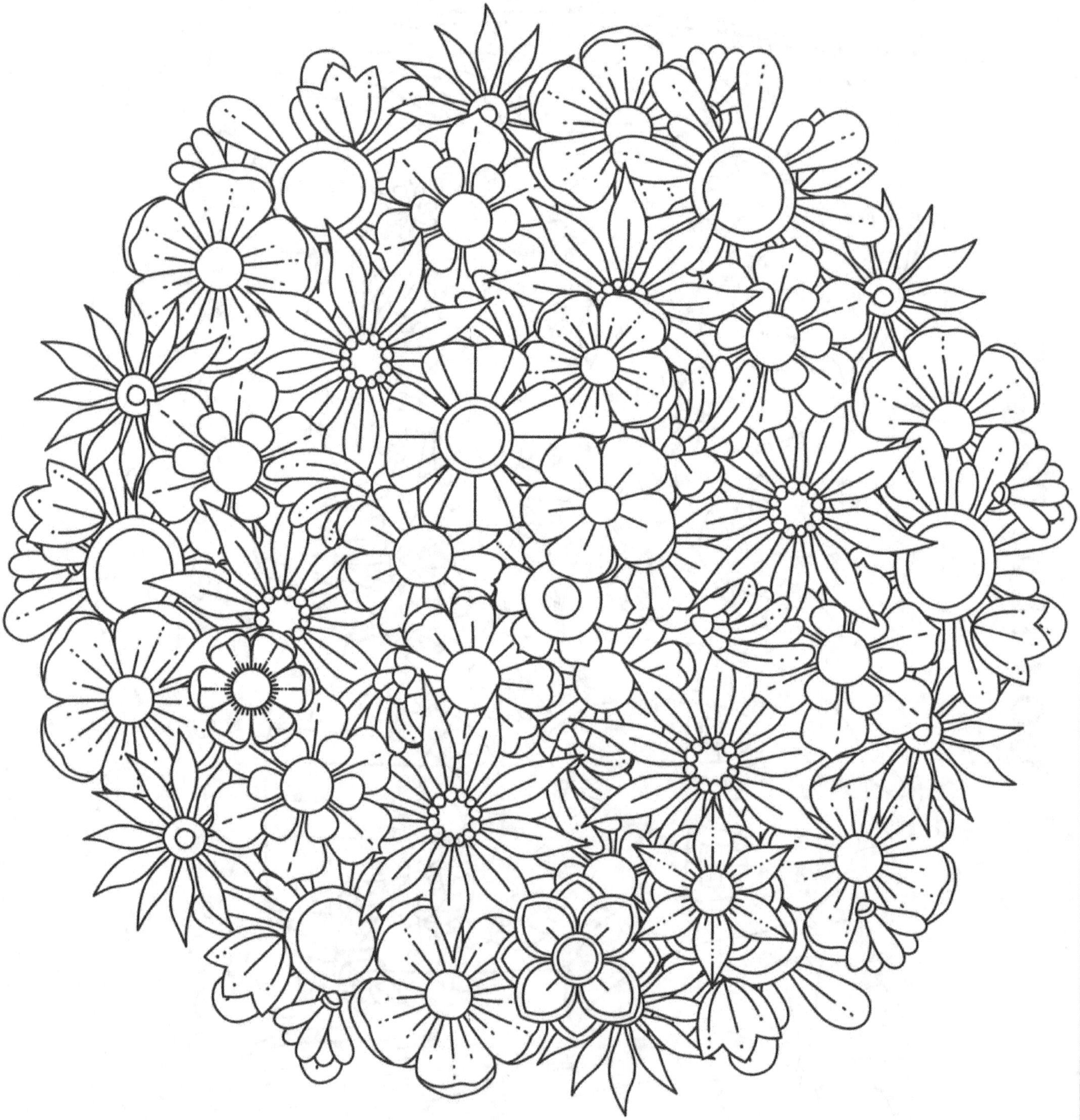

Coloring pages

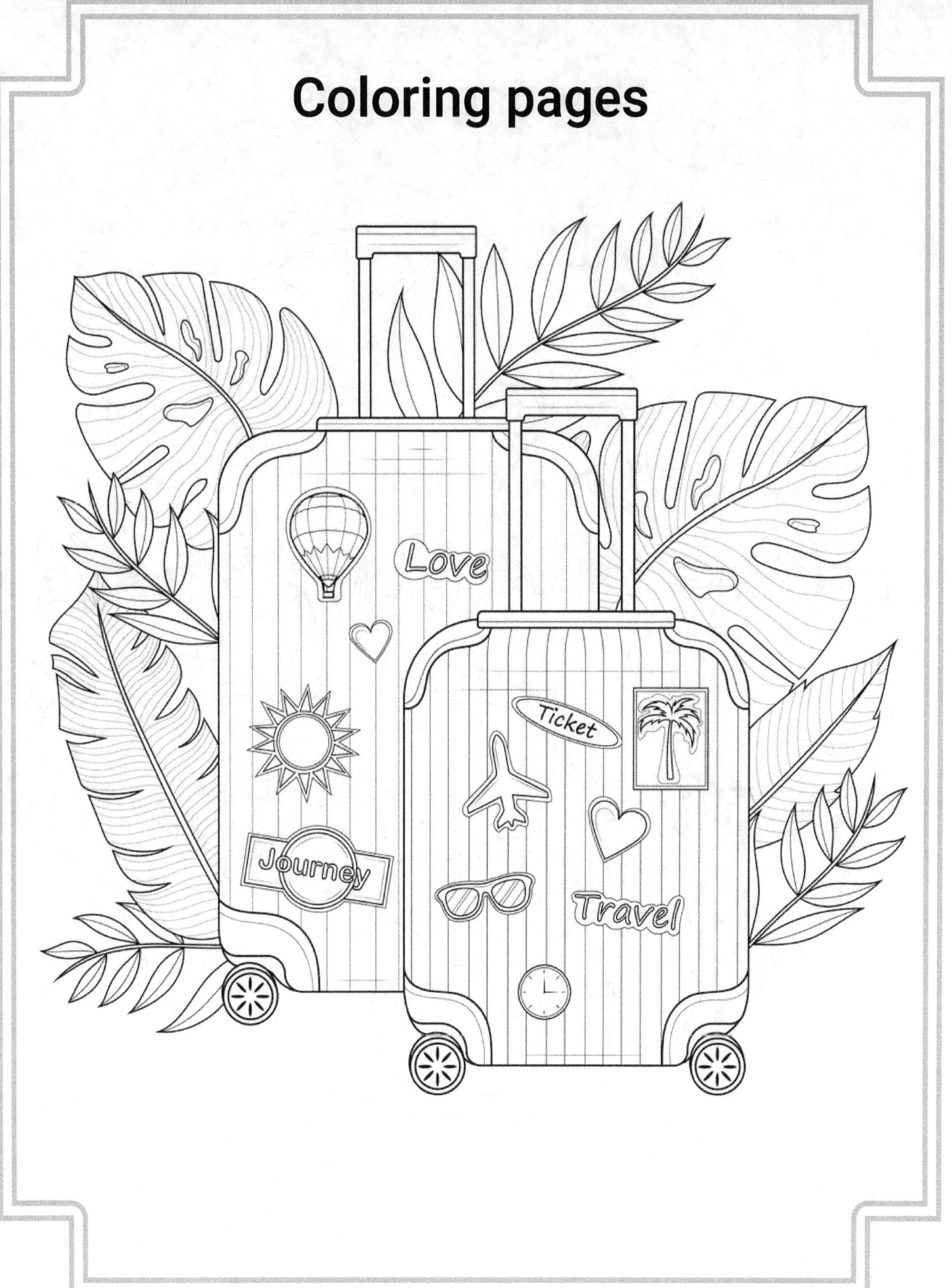

Coloring pages

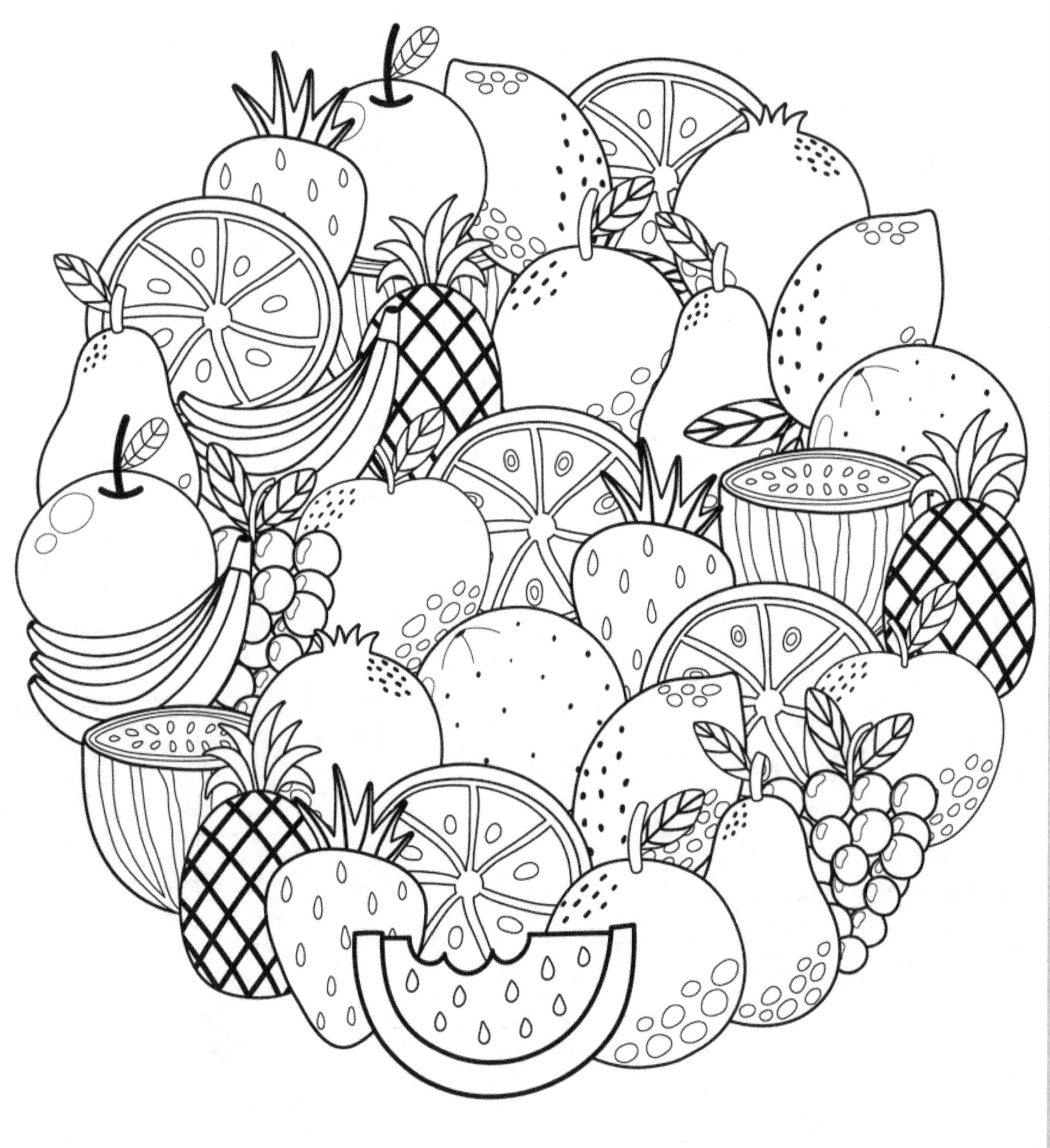

Coloring pages

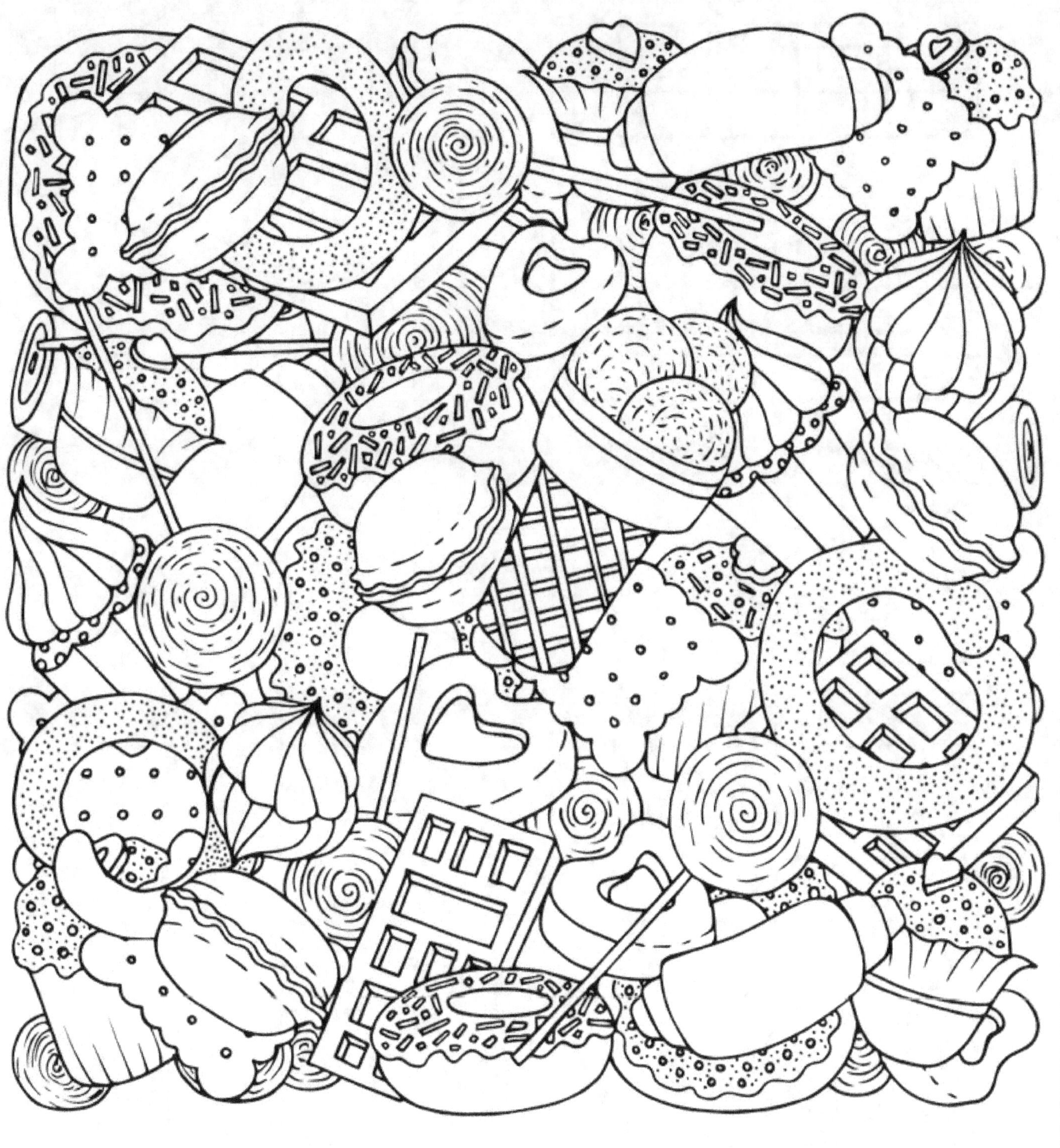

Continue the pattern

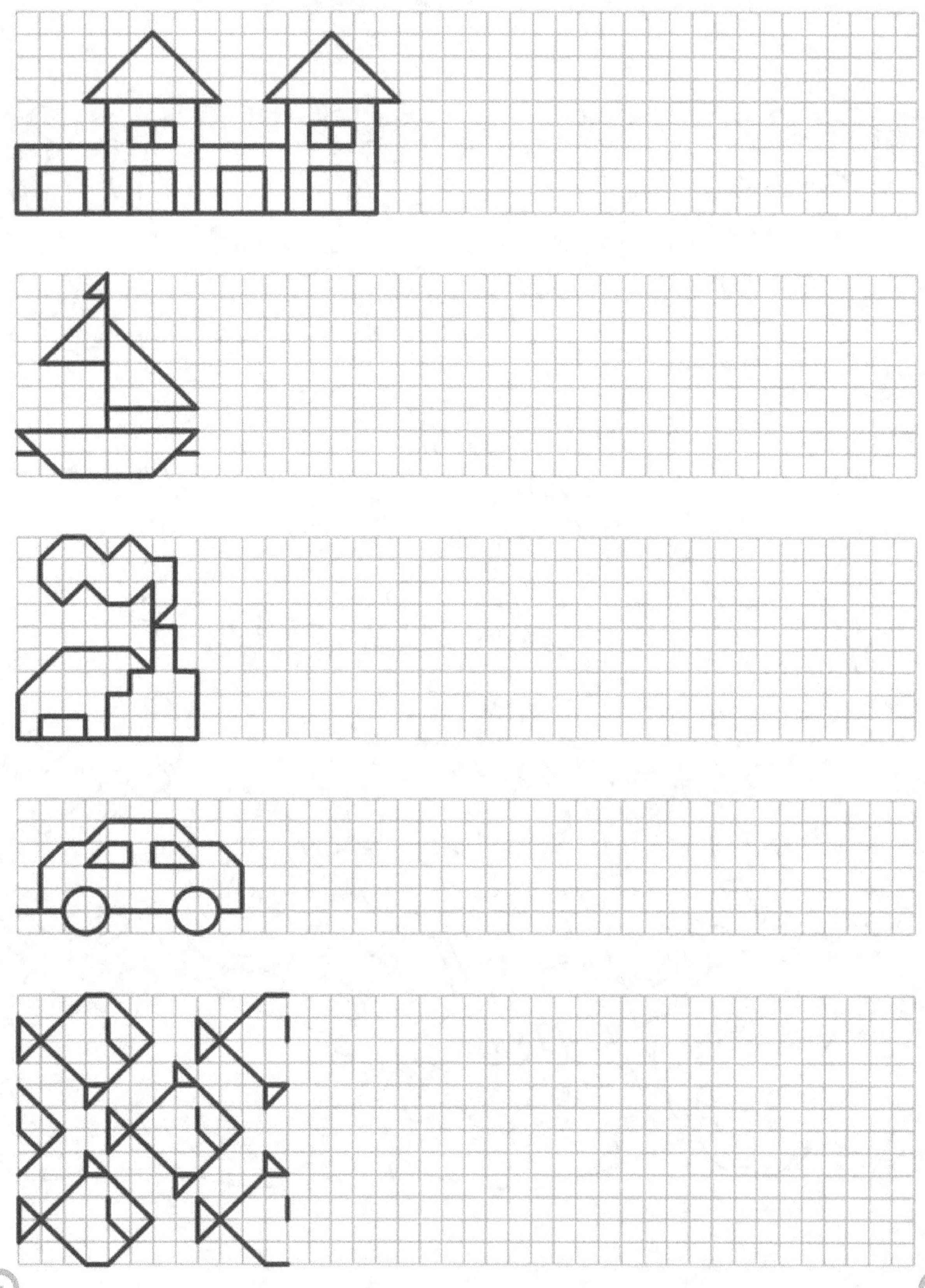

Continue the pattern

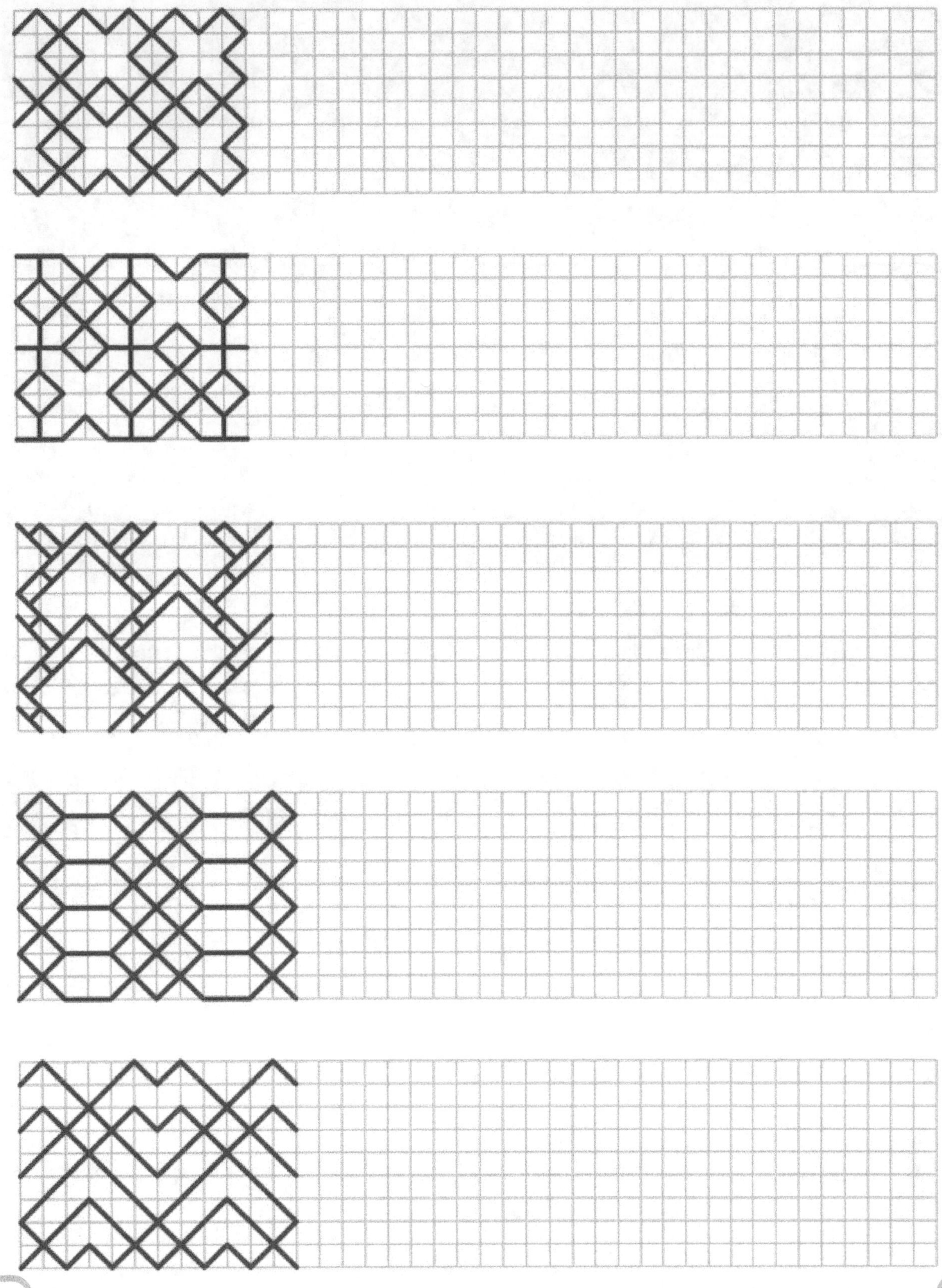

Continue the pattern

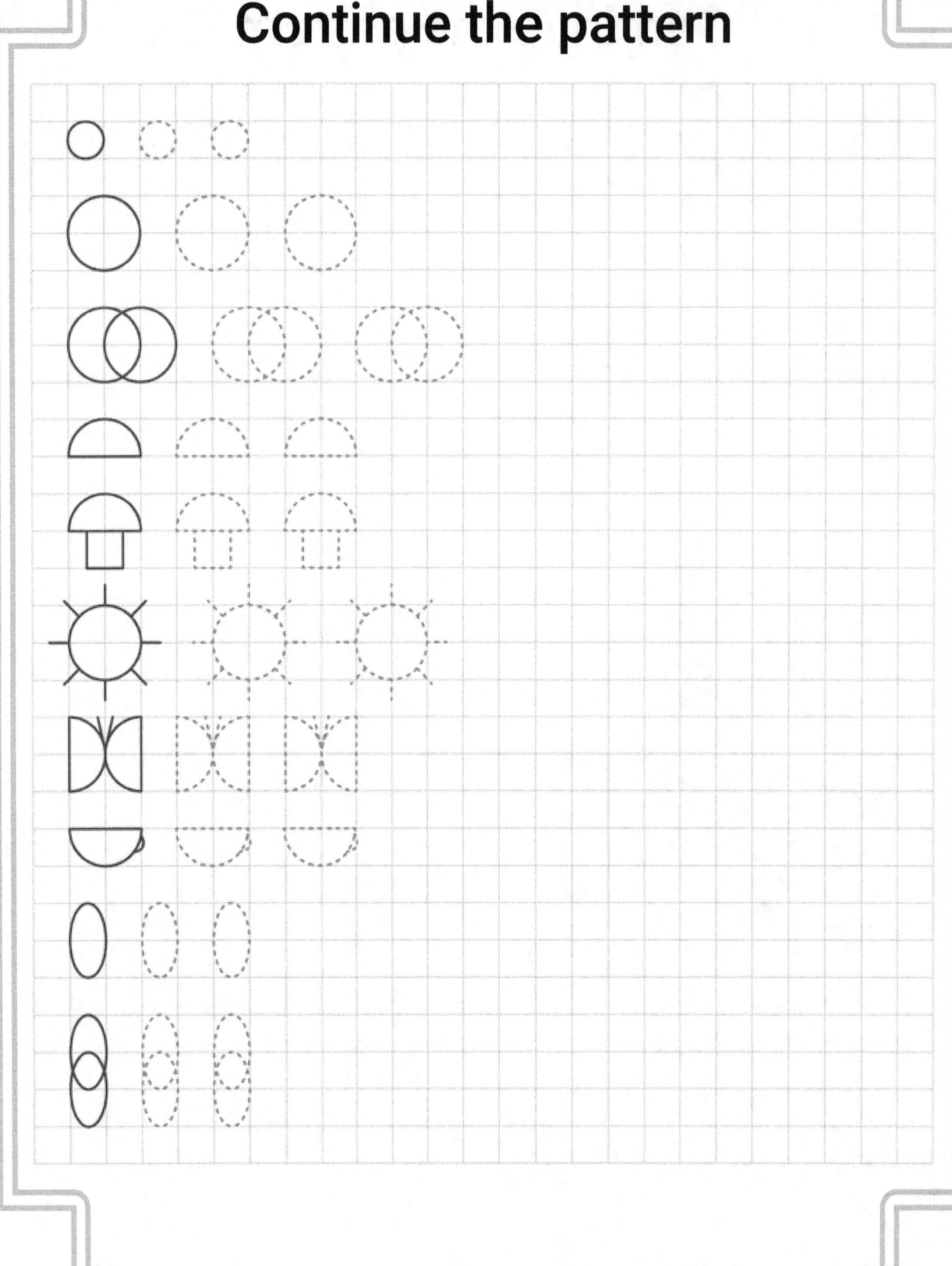

Eye-hand coordination

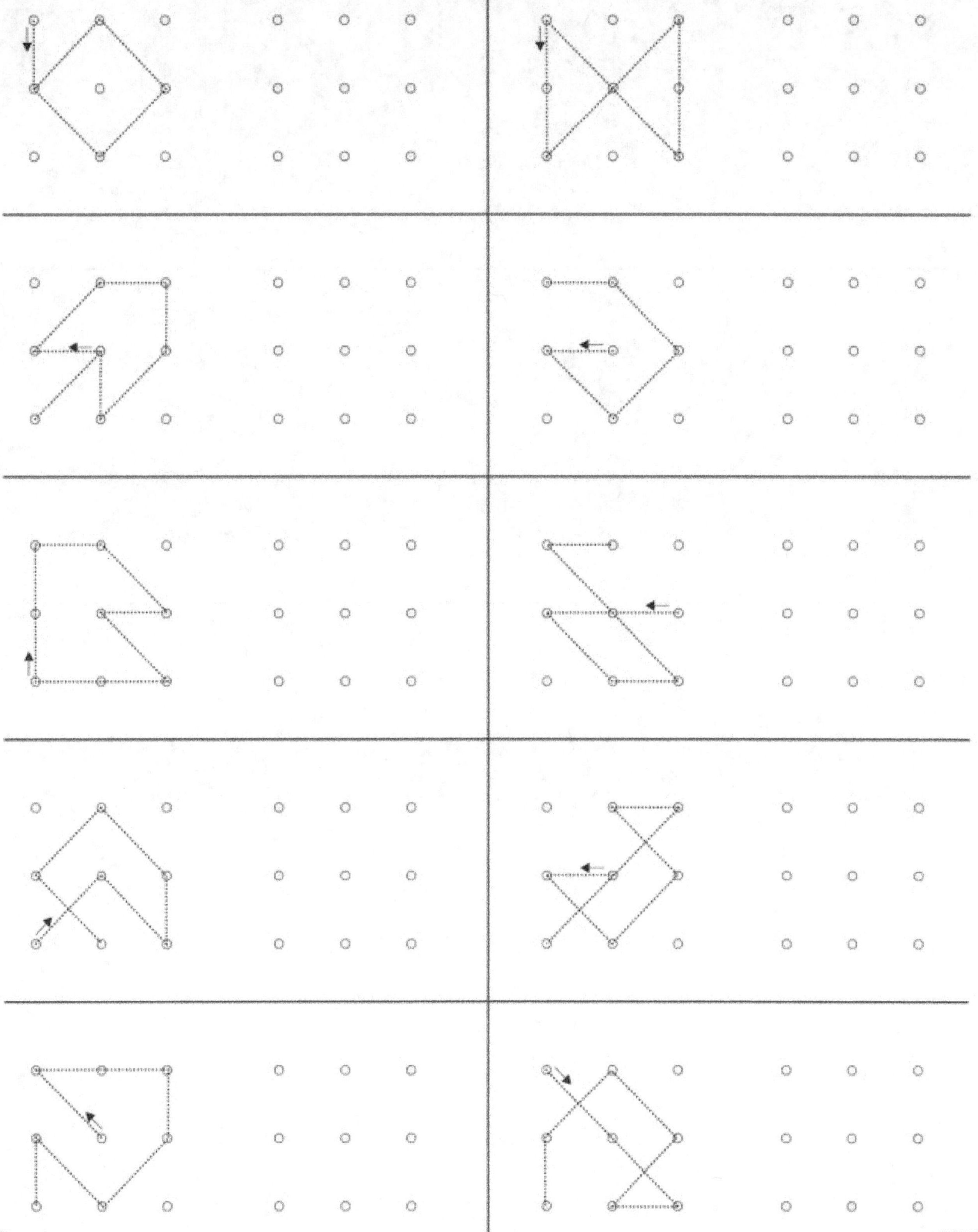

Eye-hand coordination

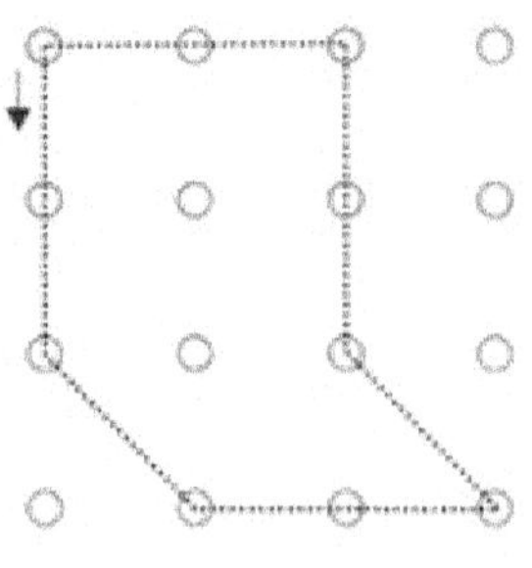 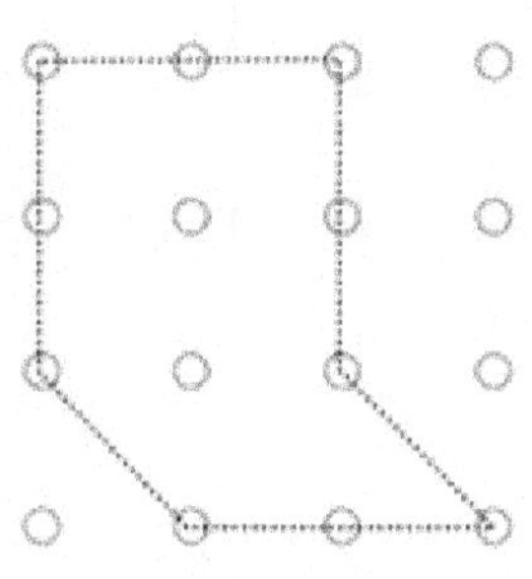 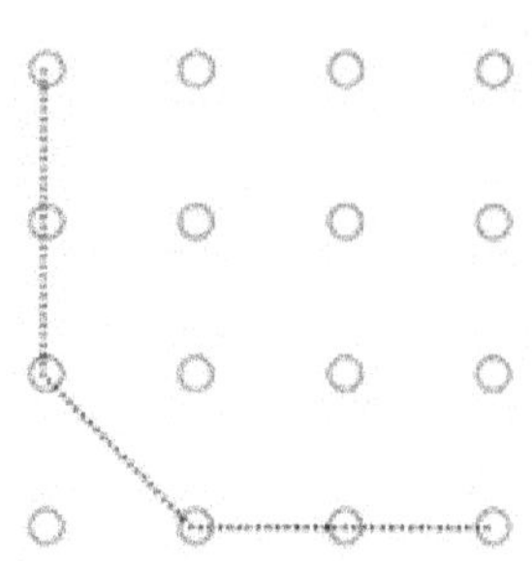

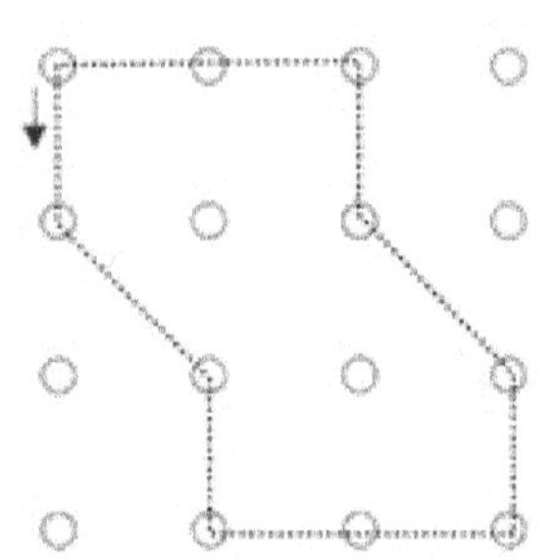 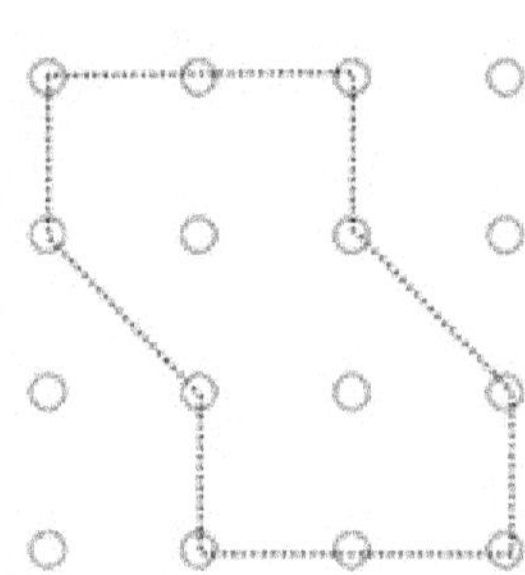 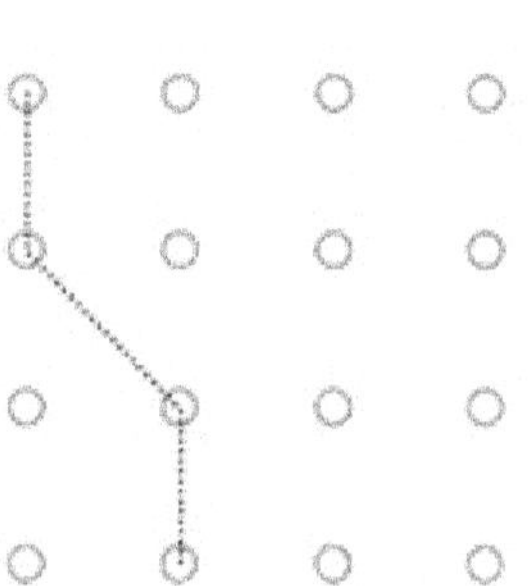

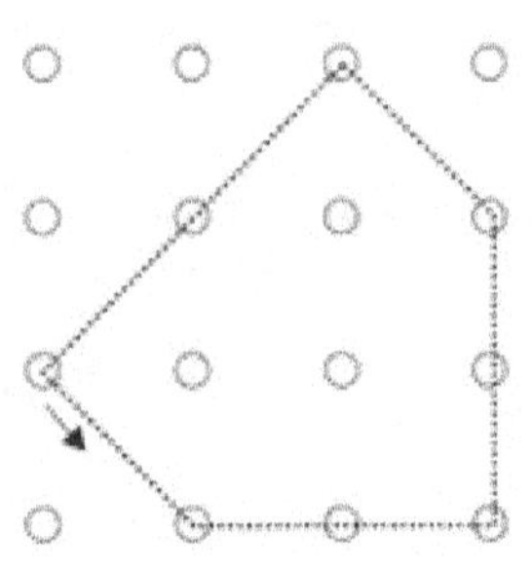 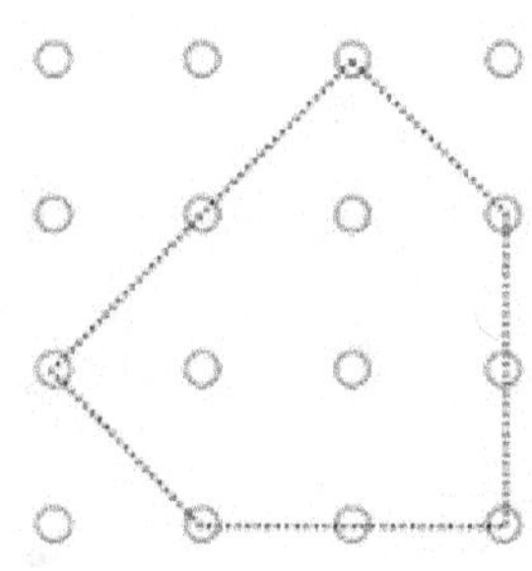 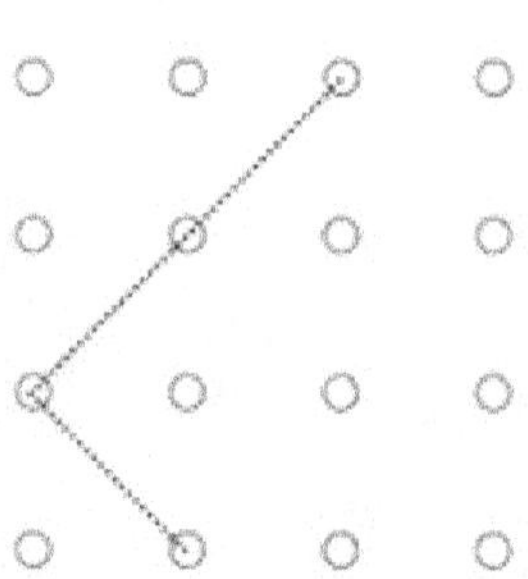

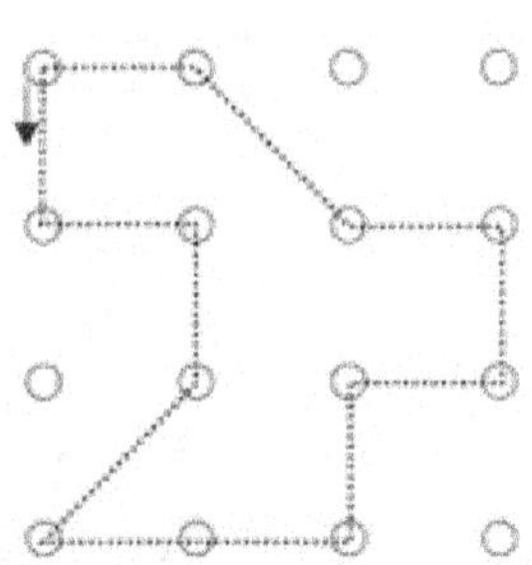 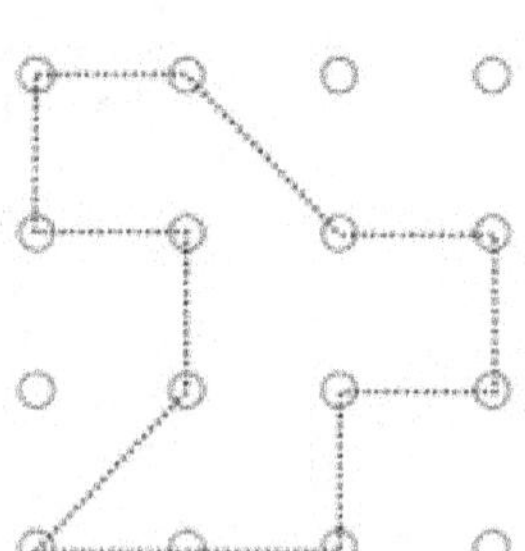 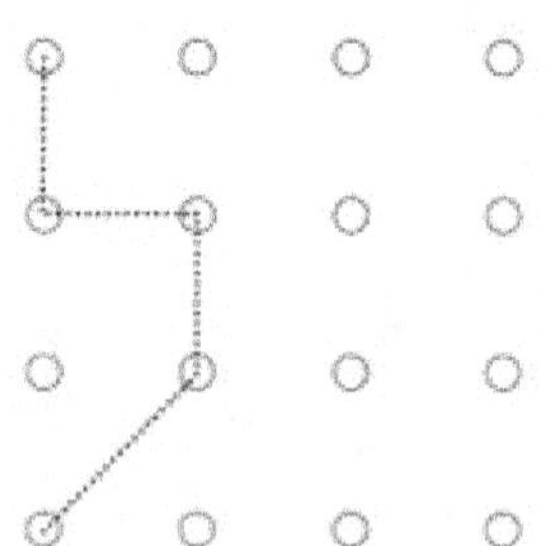

Eye-hand coordination

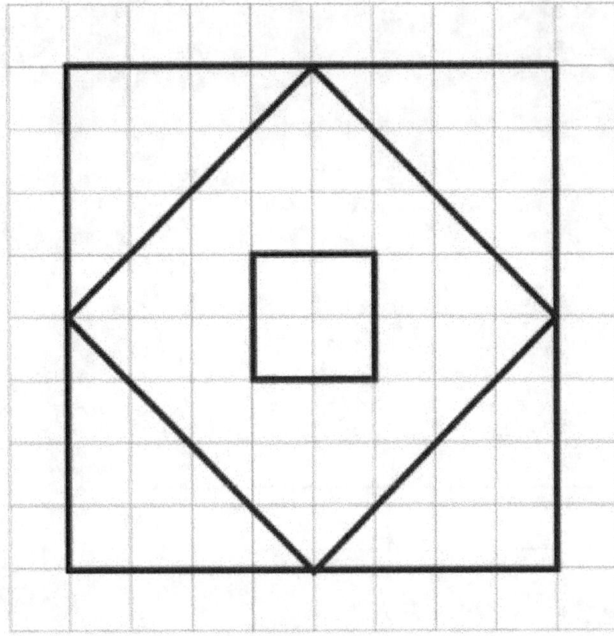

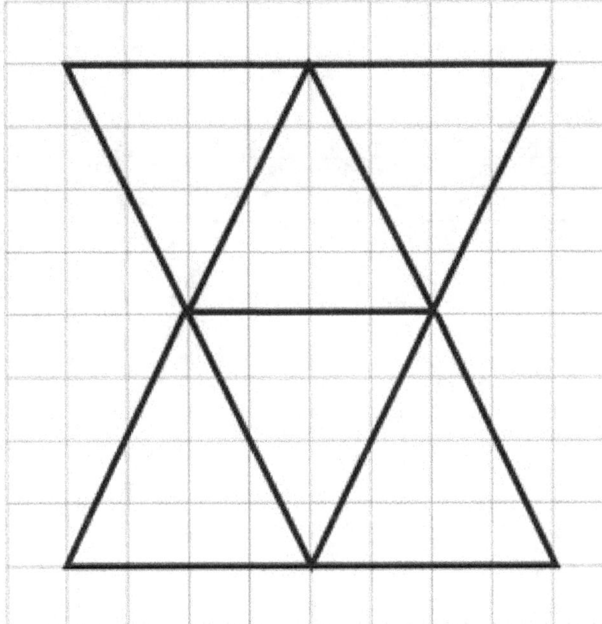

Eye-hand coordination

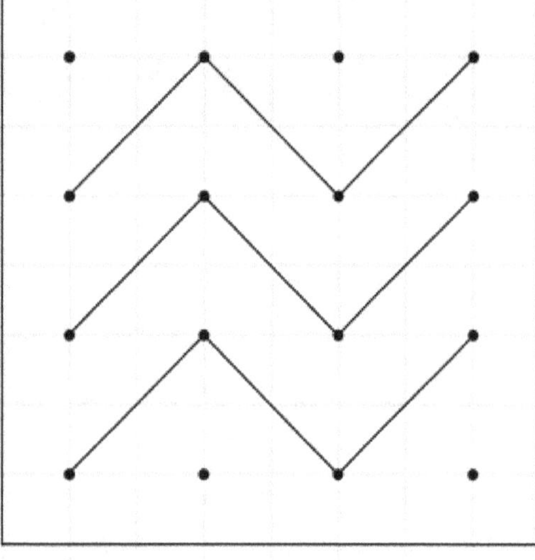 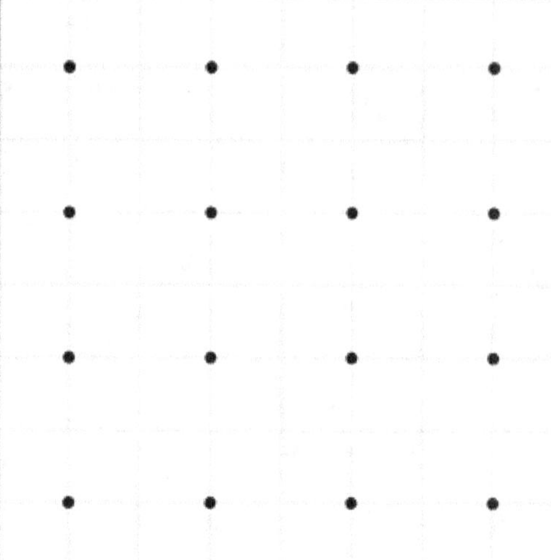

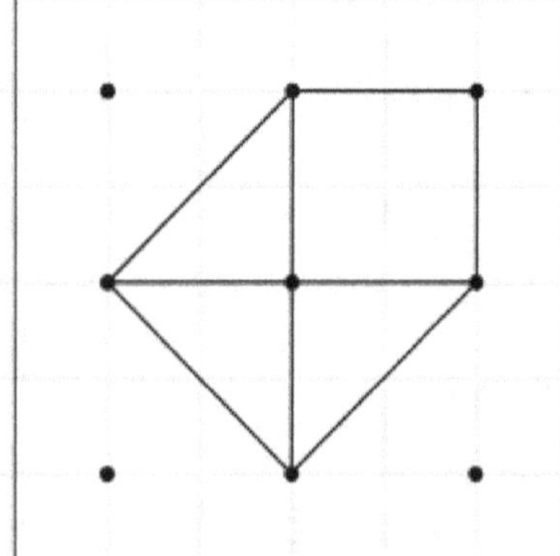 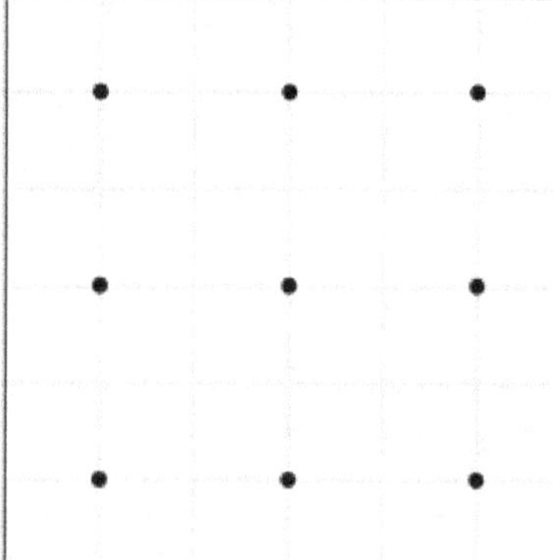

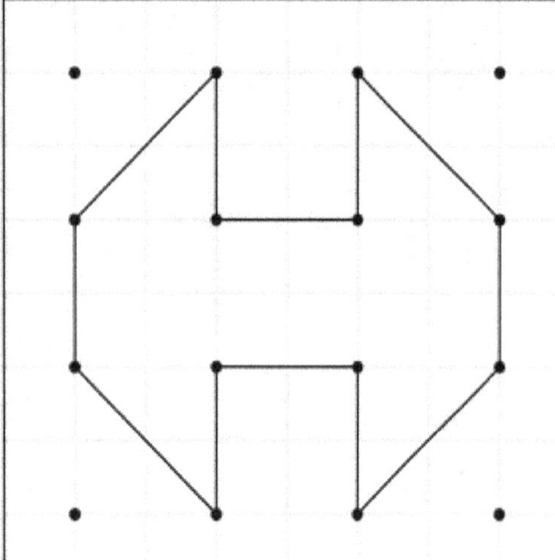 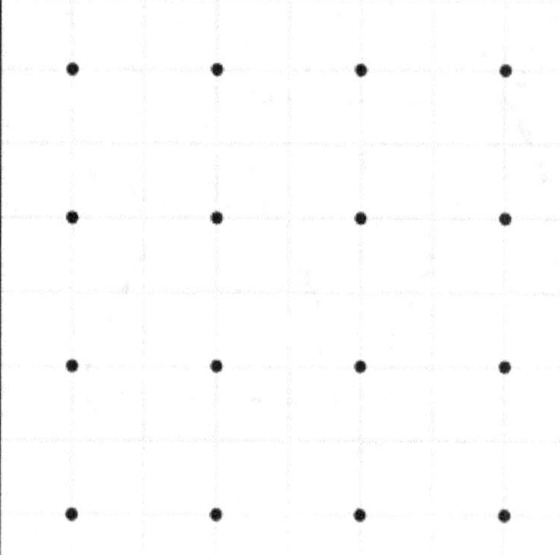

Eye-hand coordination

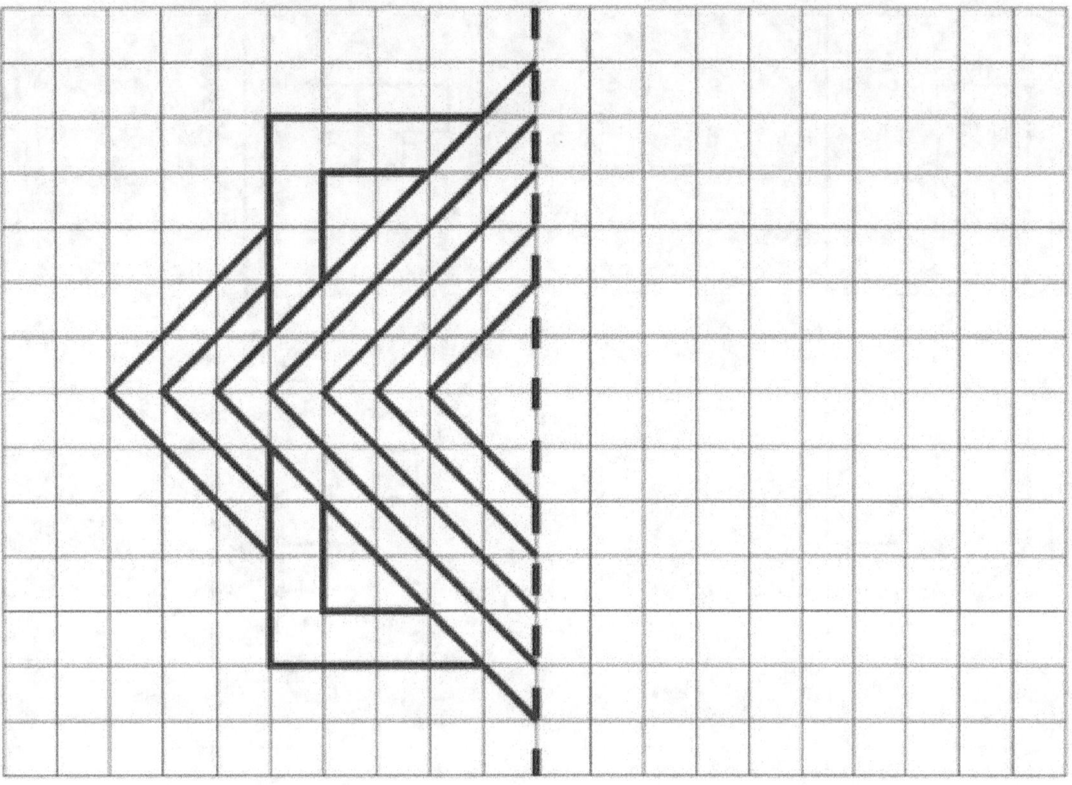

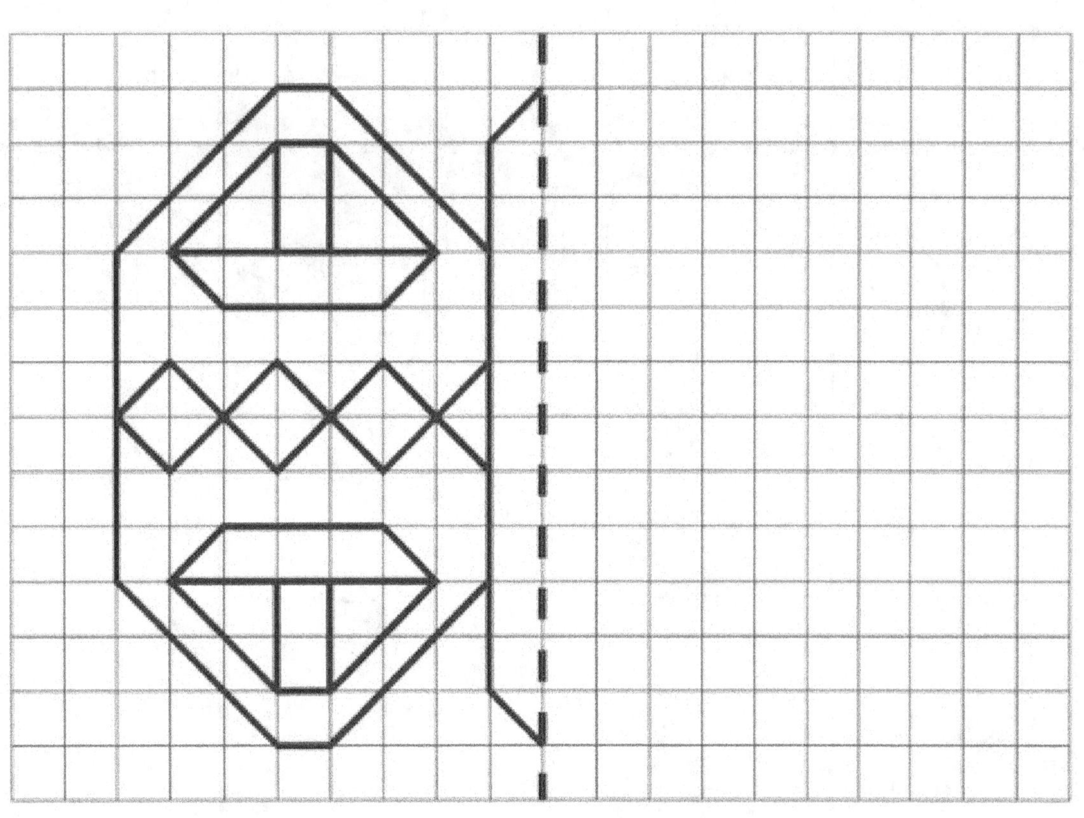

Eye-hand coordination

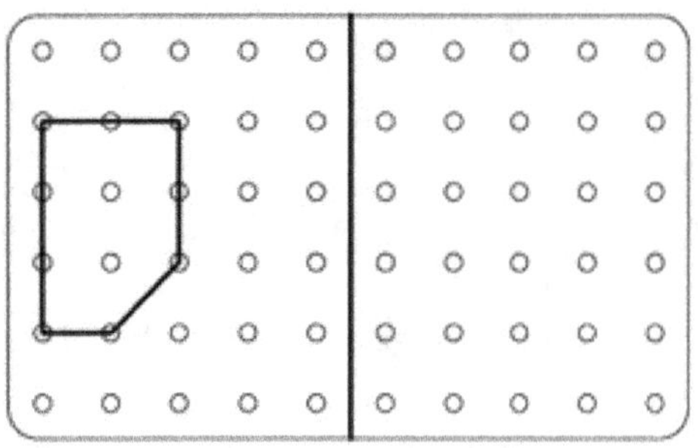
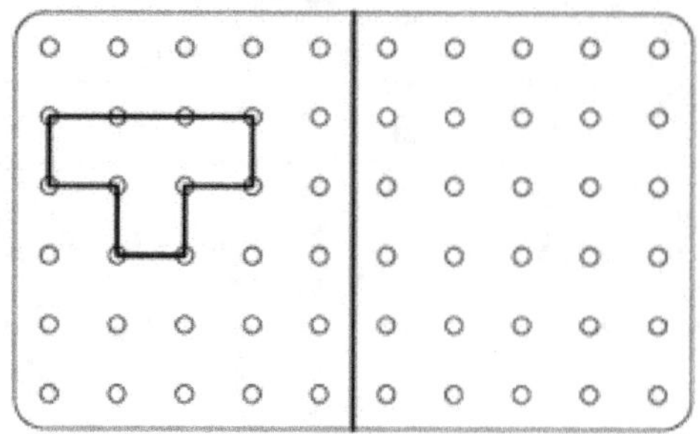

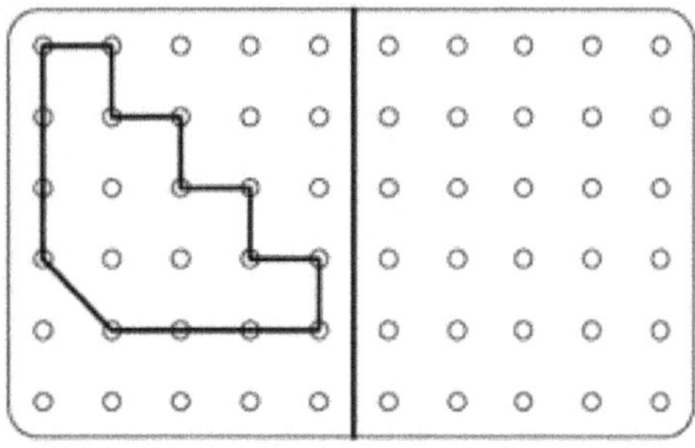
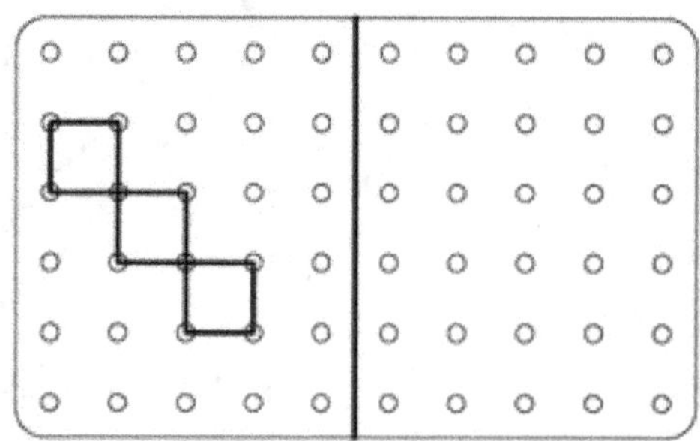

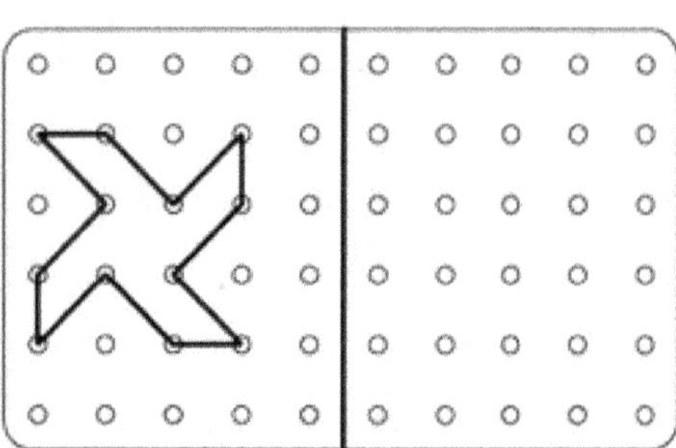
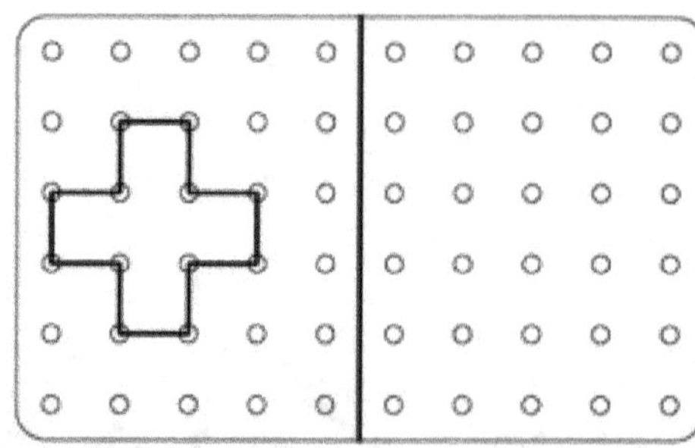

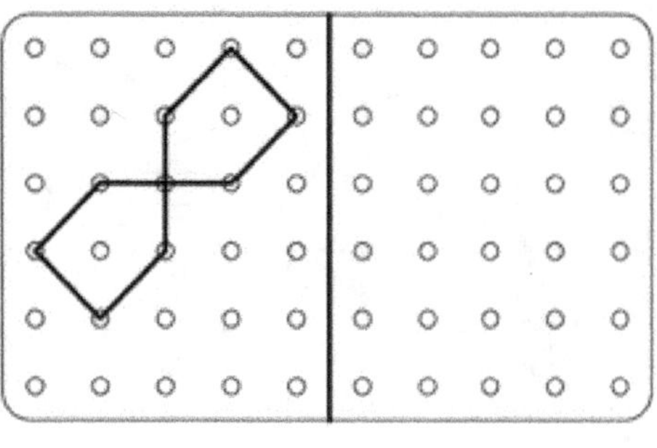
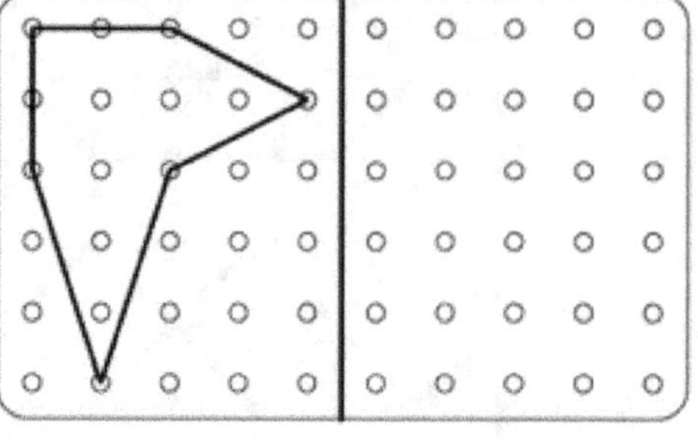

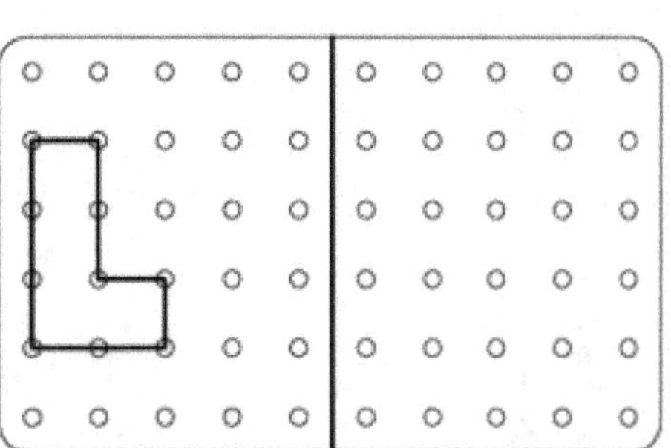
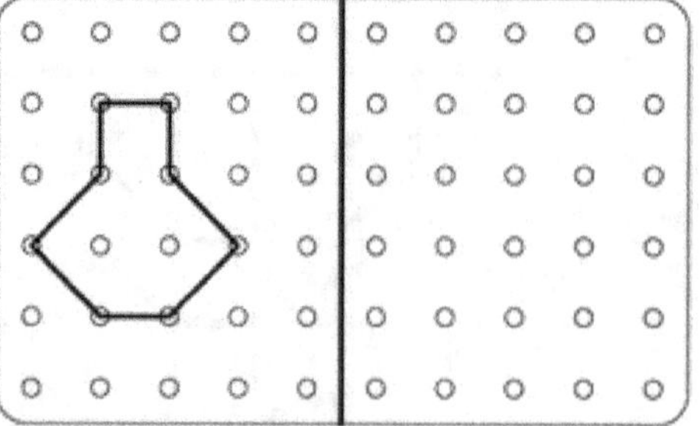

Find the ten differences between the two pictures.

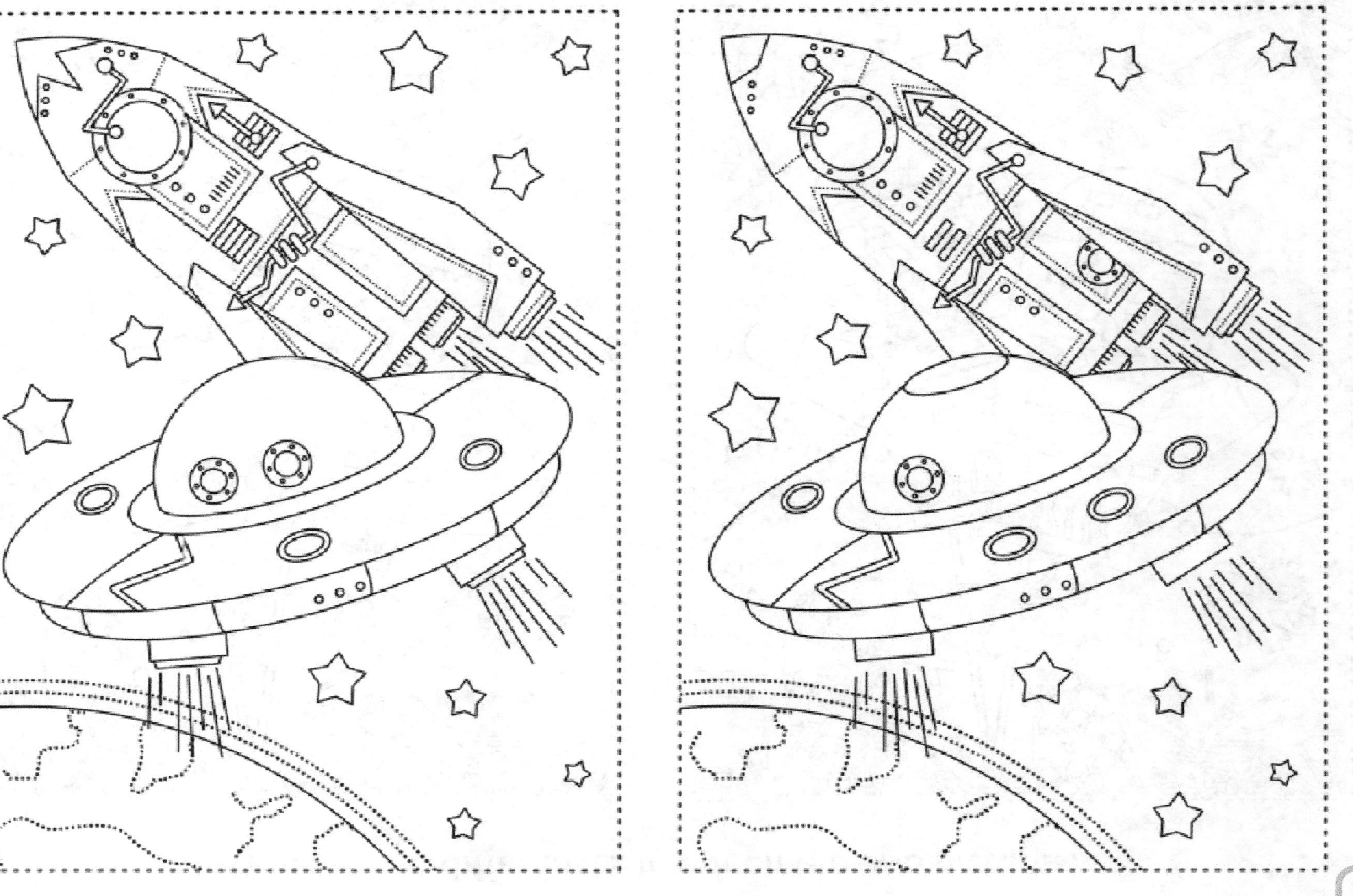

Find the ten differences between the two pictures.

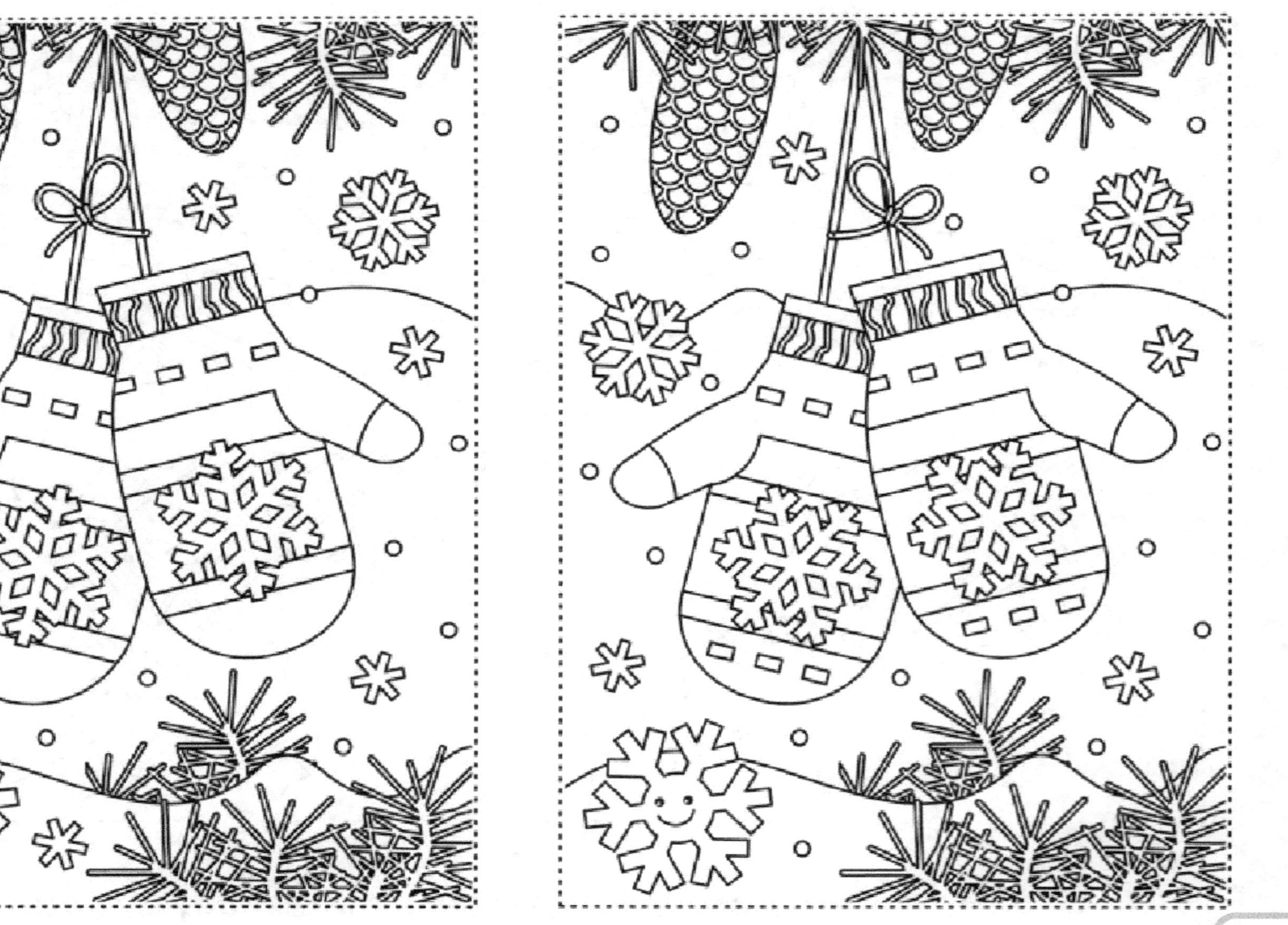

Find the ten differences between the two pictures.

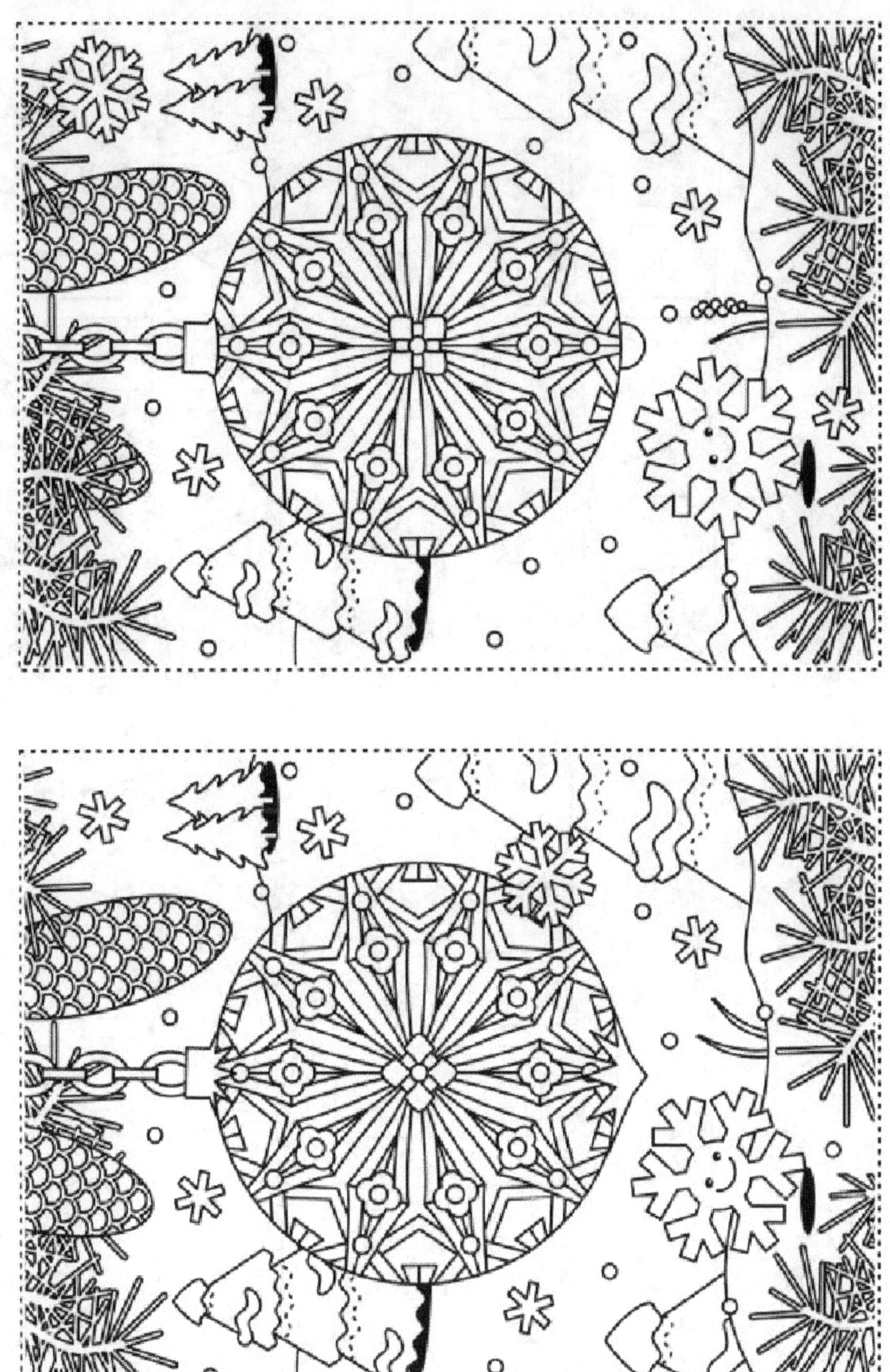

Find 10 differences.

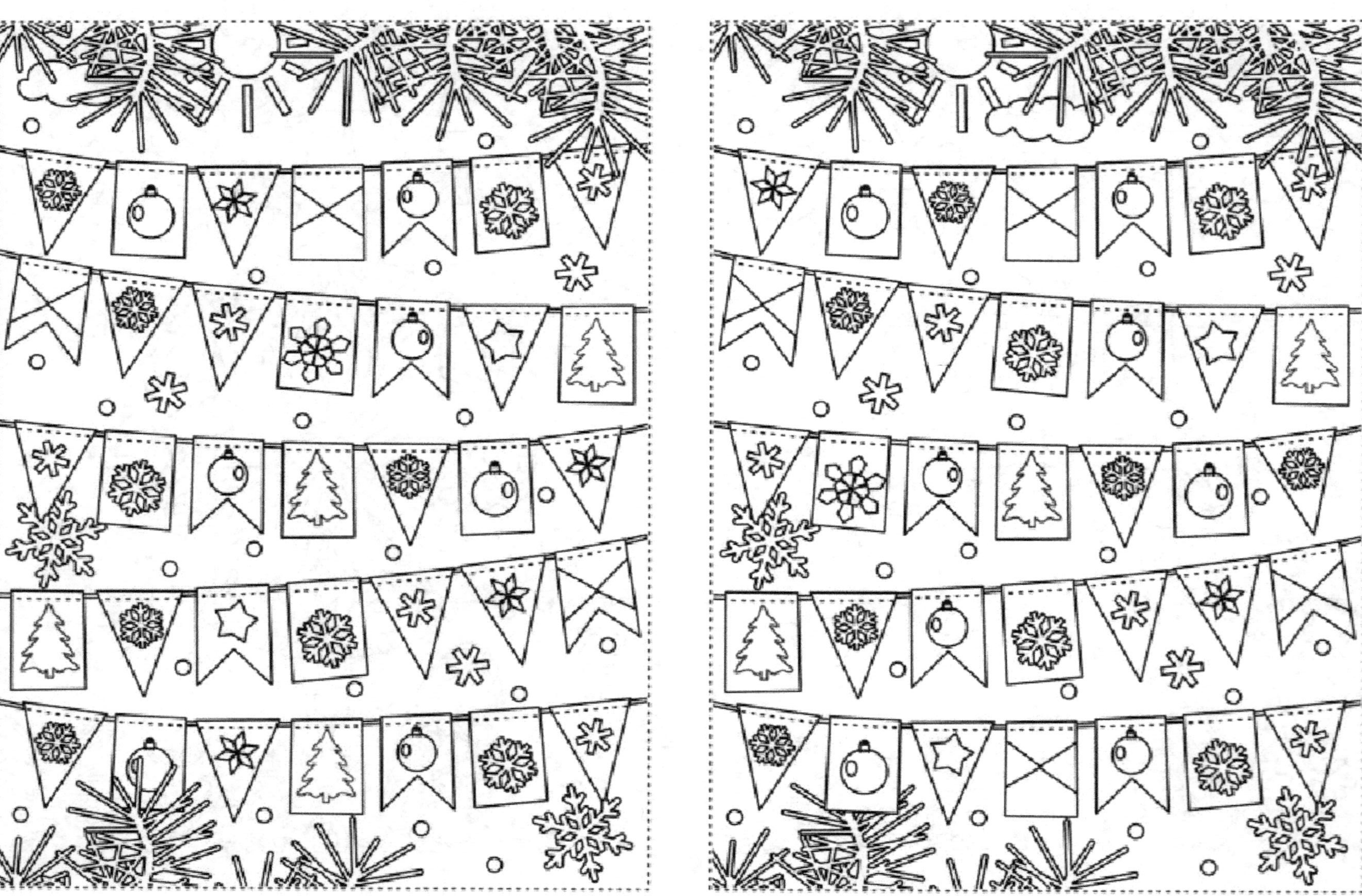

Find 10 differences.

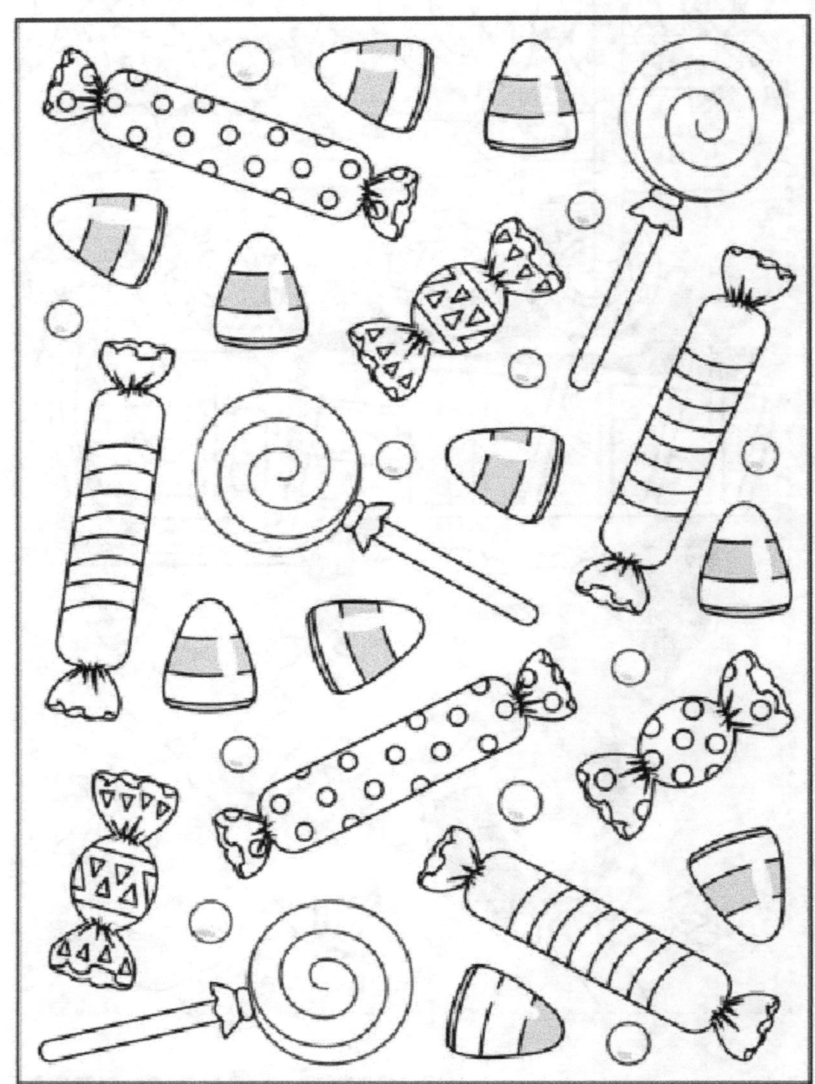

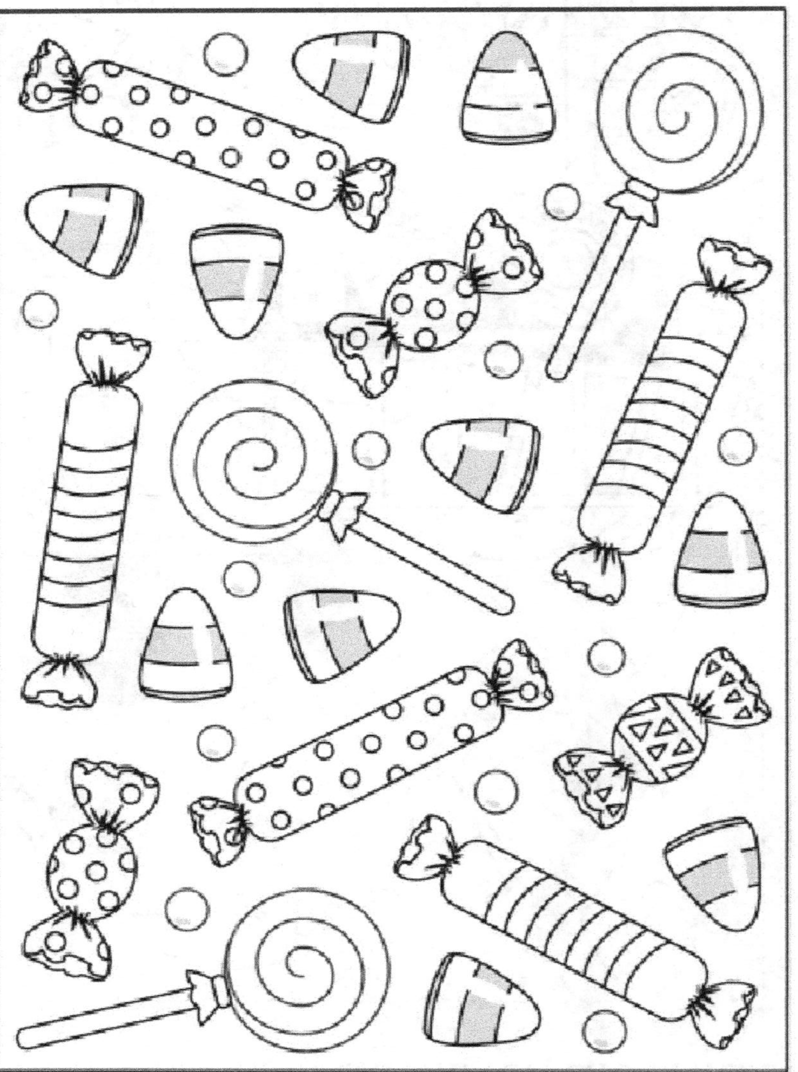

Find the ten differences between the two pictures.

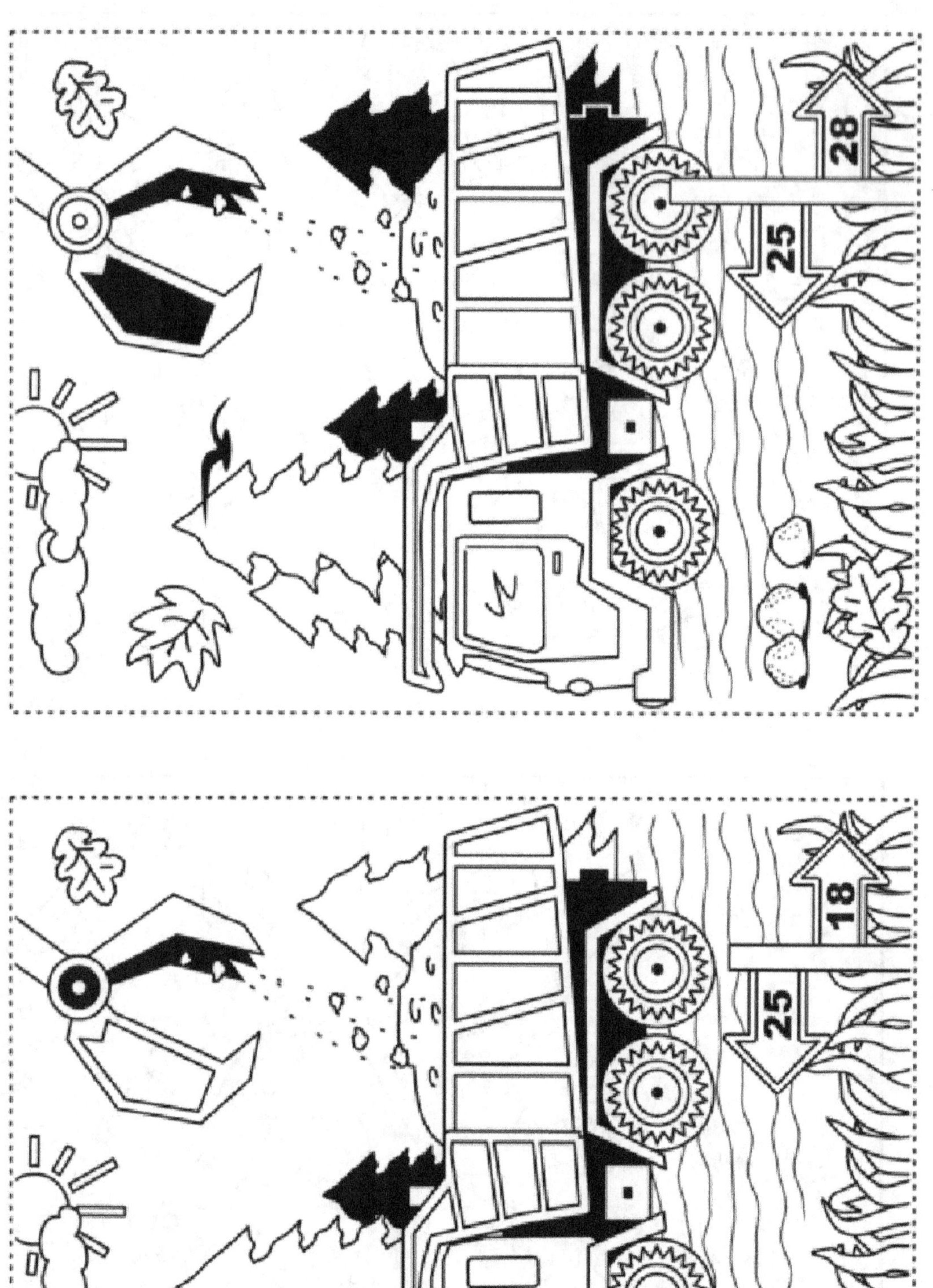

Find 5 differences

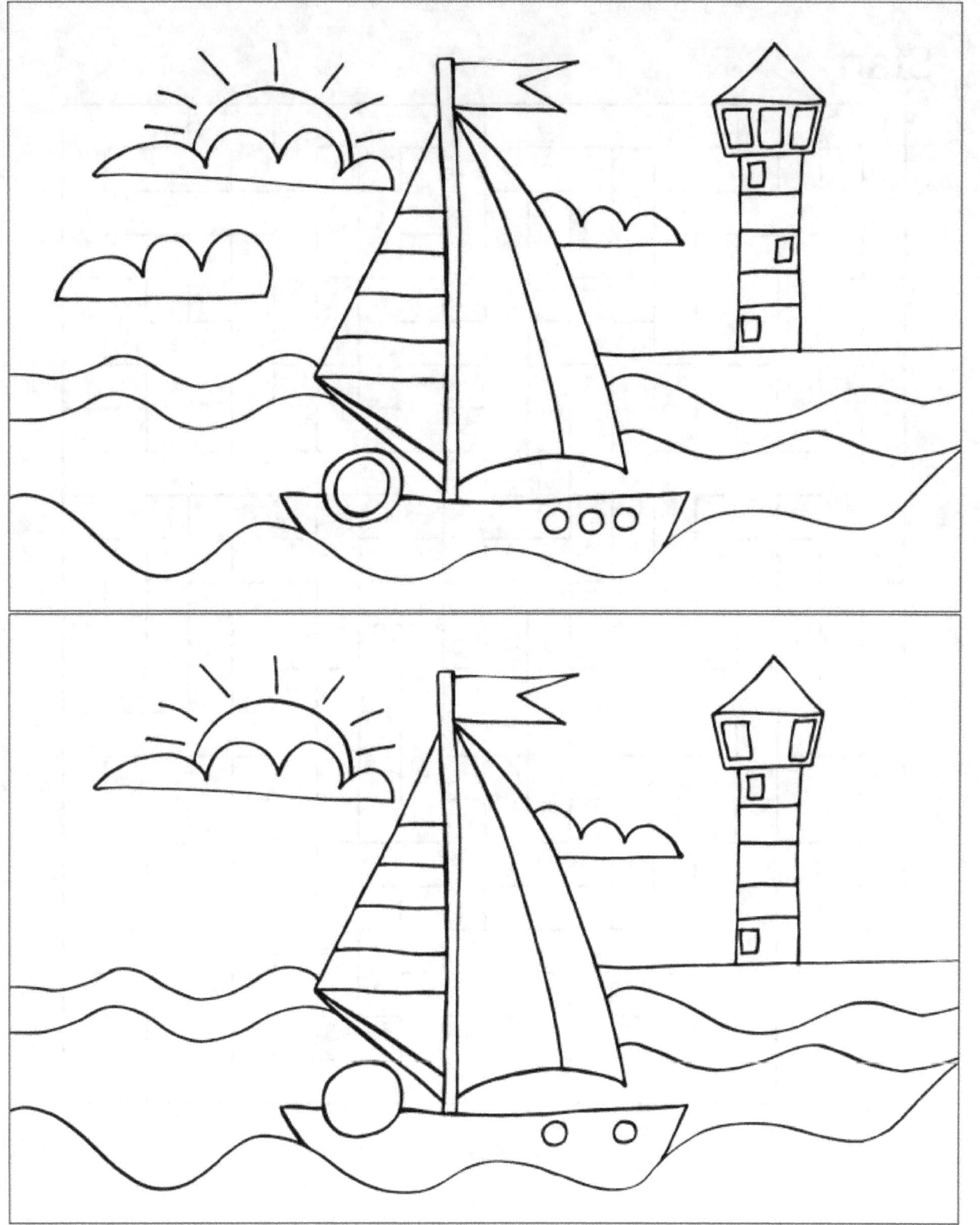

Maze 1

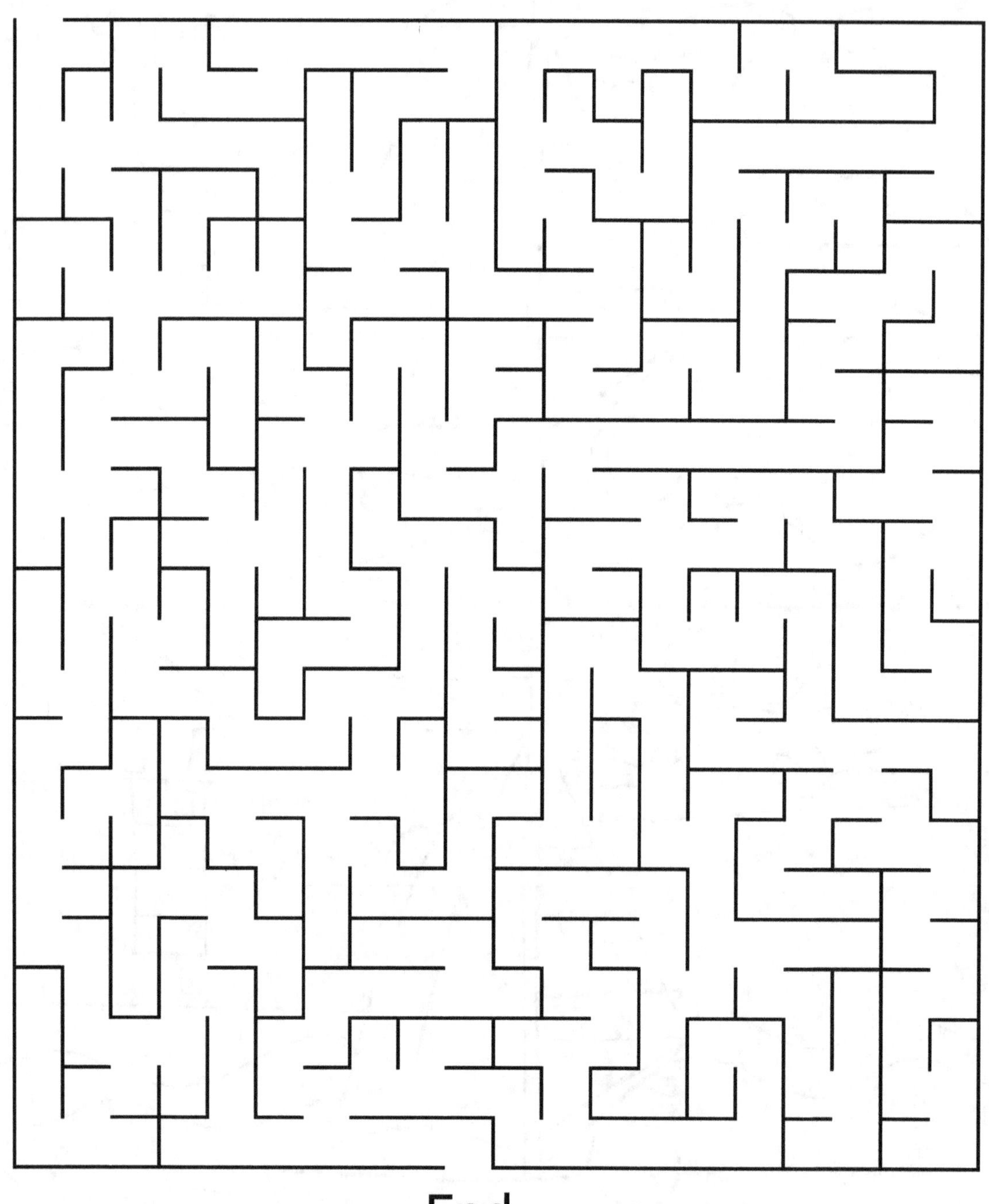

Maze 2

Maze 3

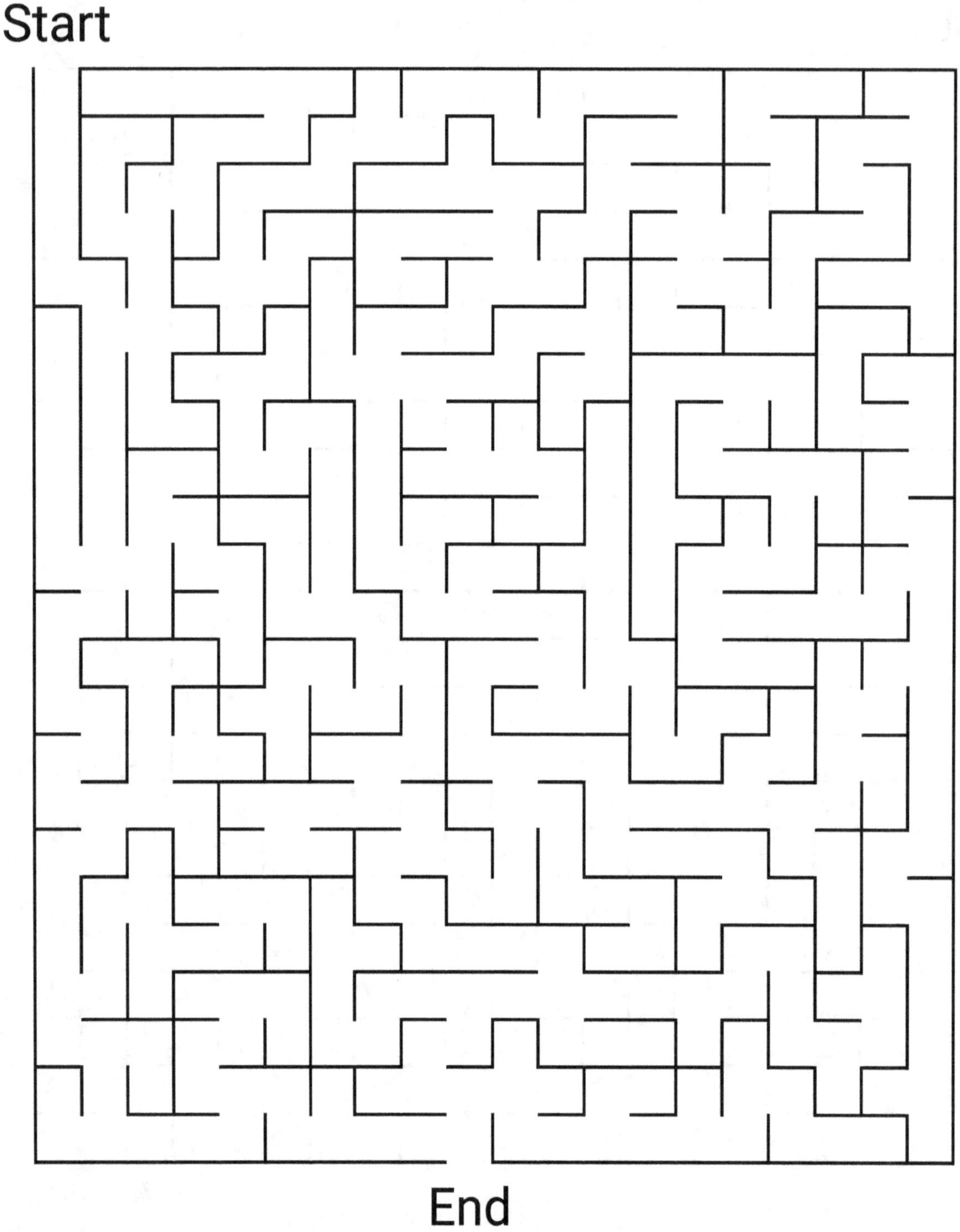

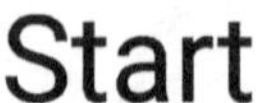

Start

End

Maze 4

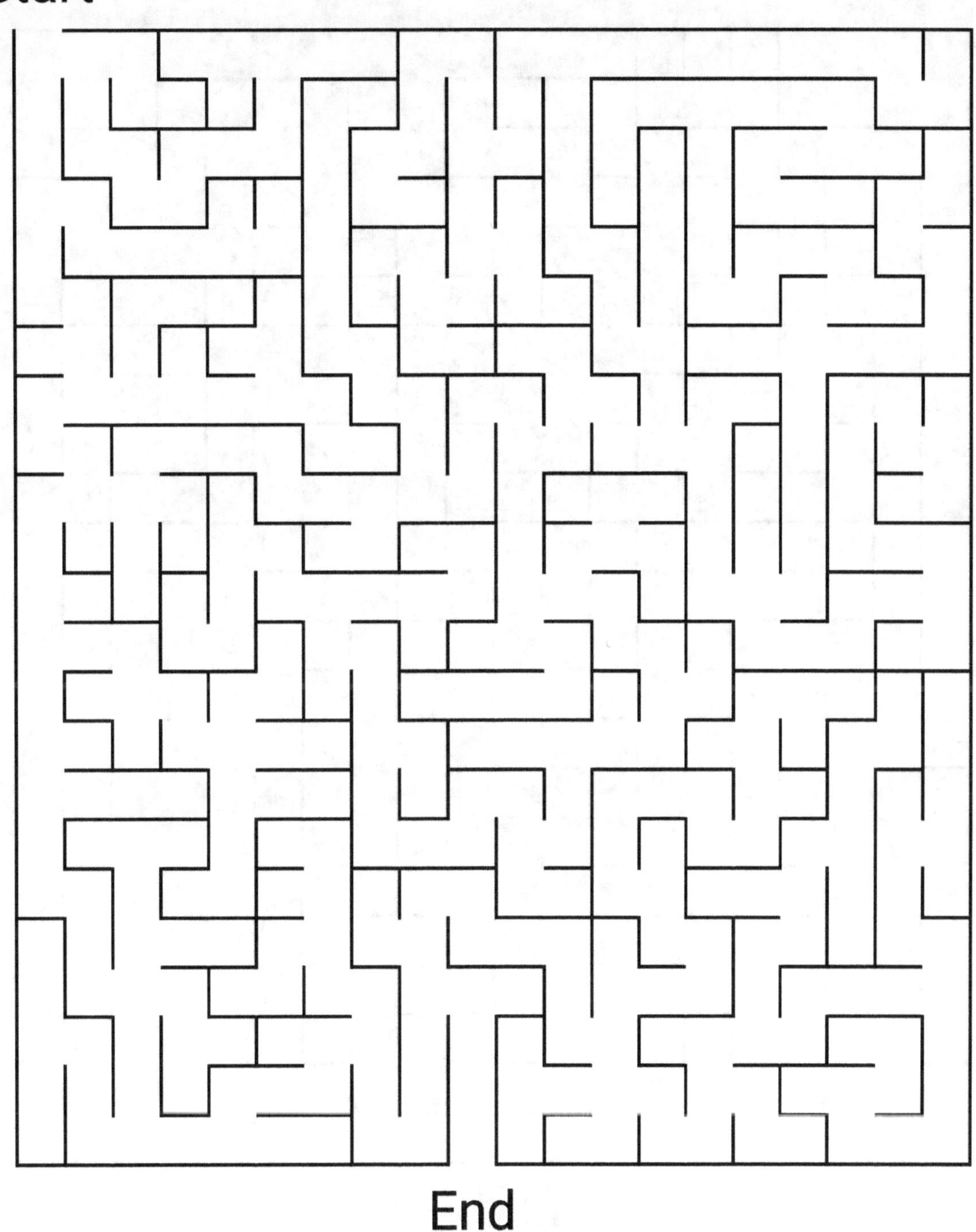

Maze 5

Start

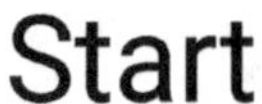

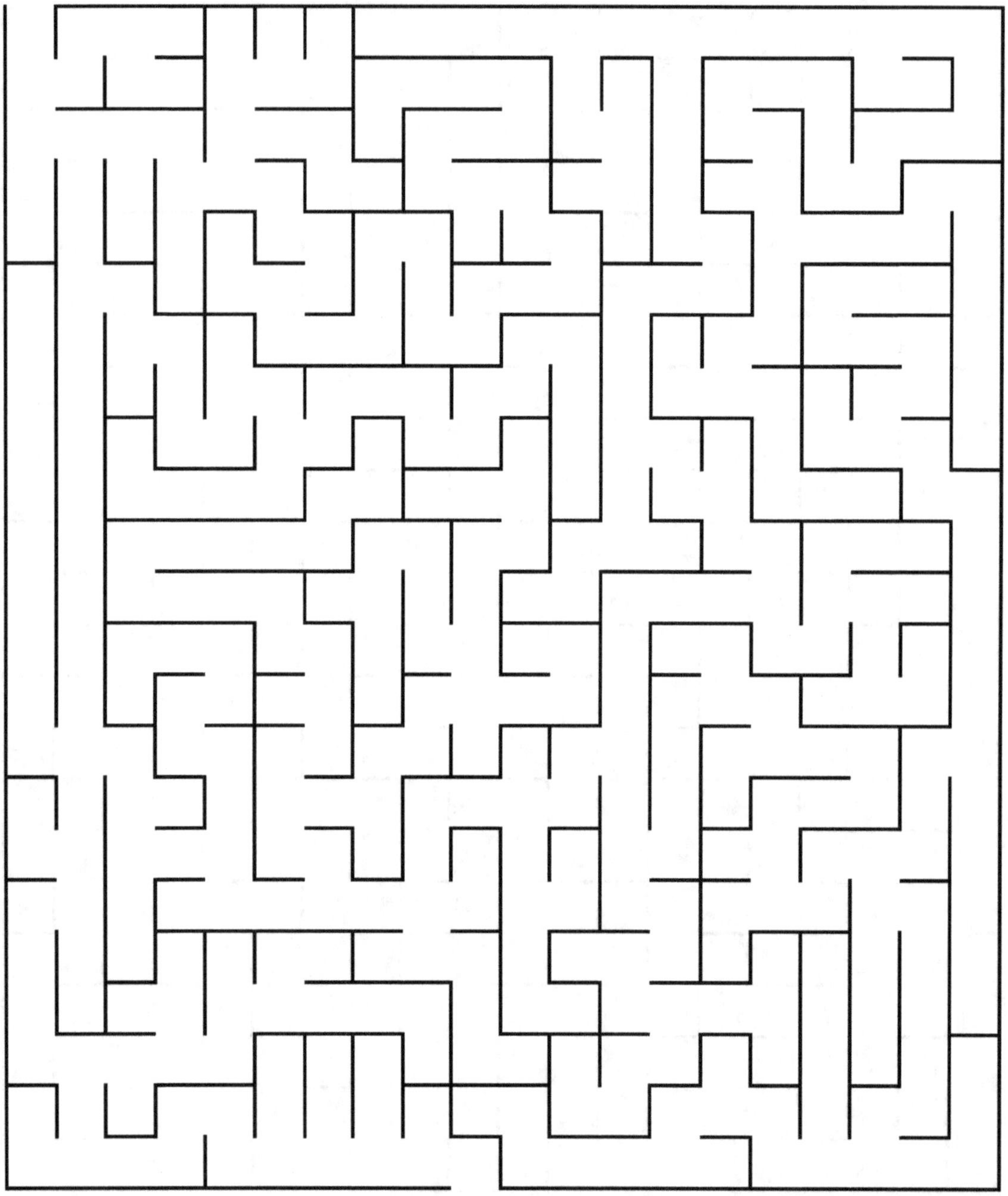

End

Maze 6

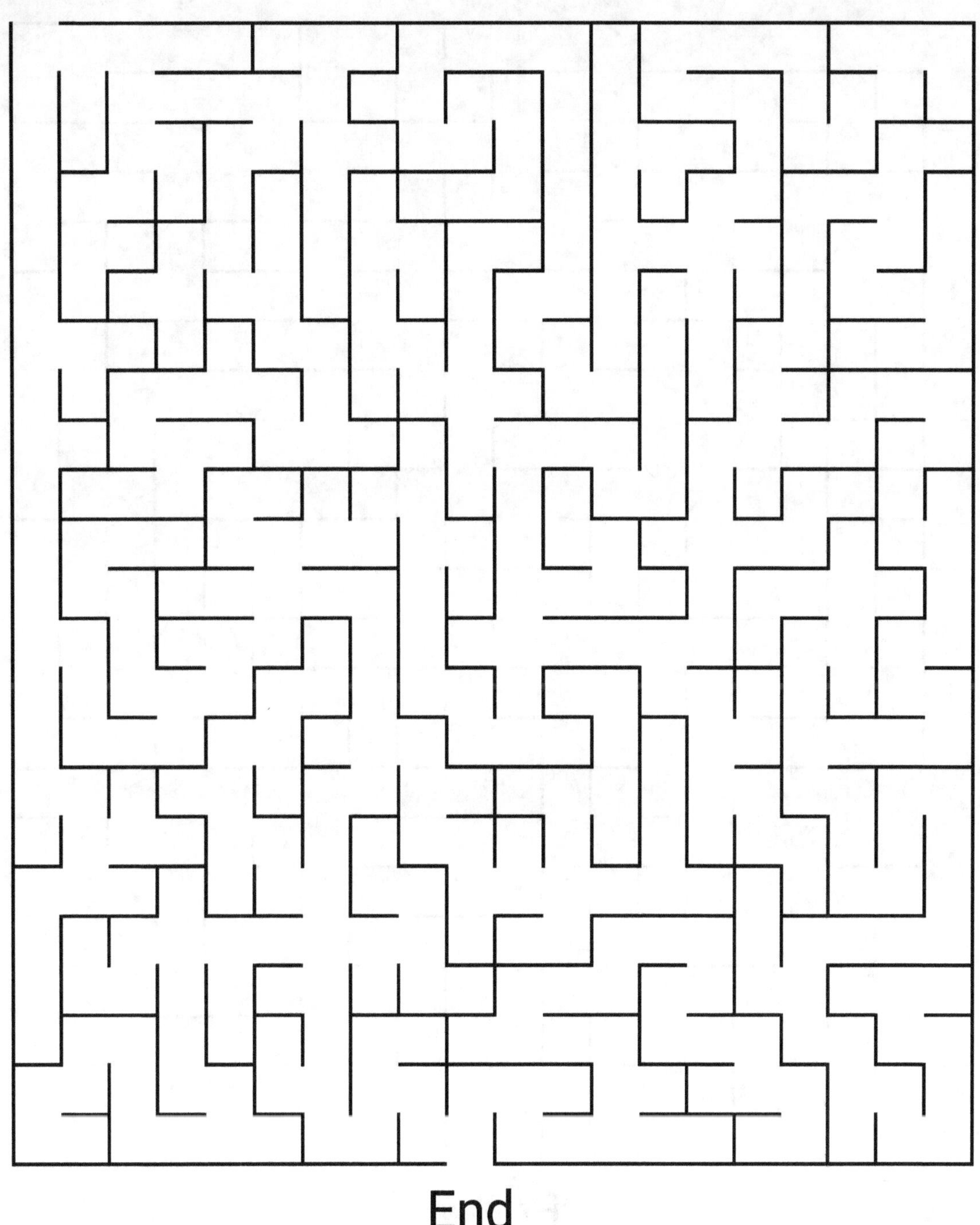

Maze 7

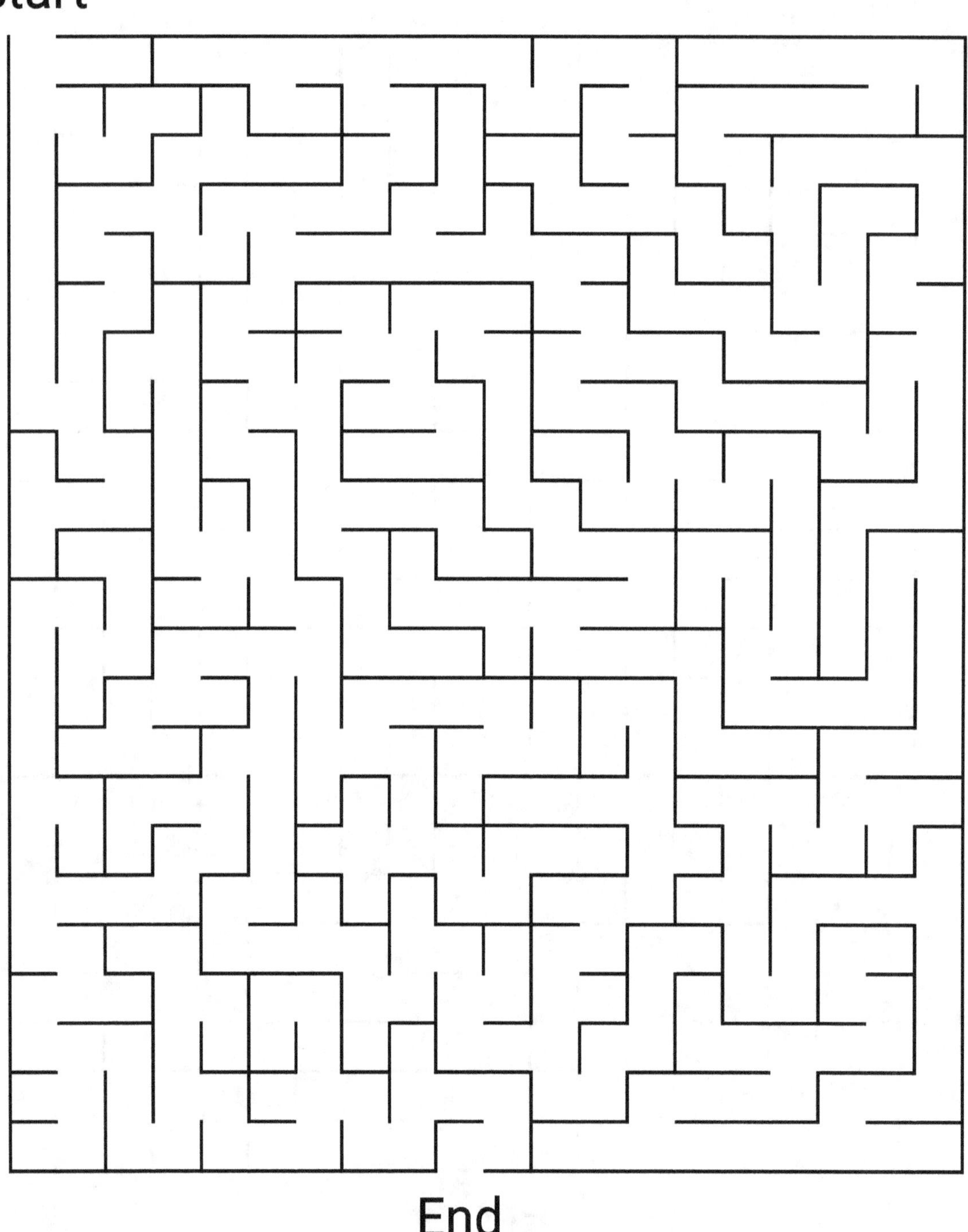

Maze 8

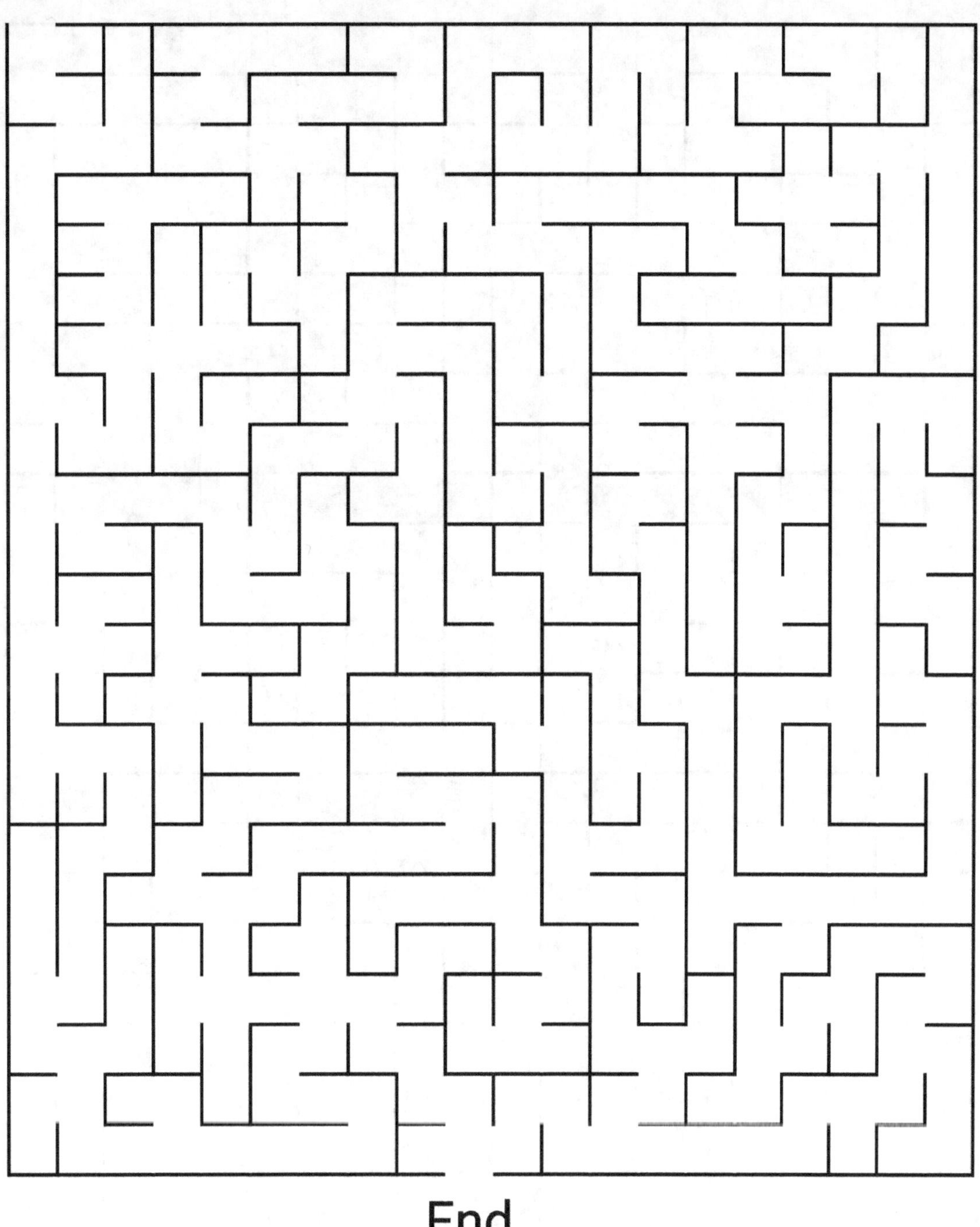

Maze 9

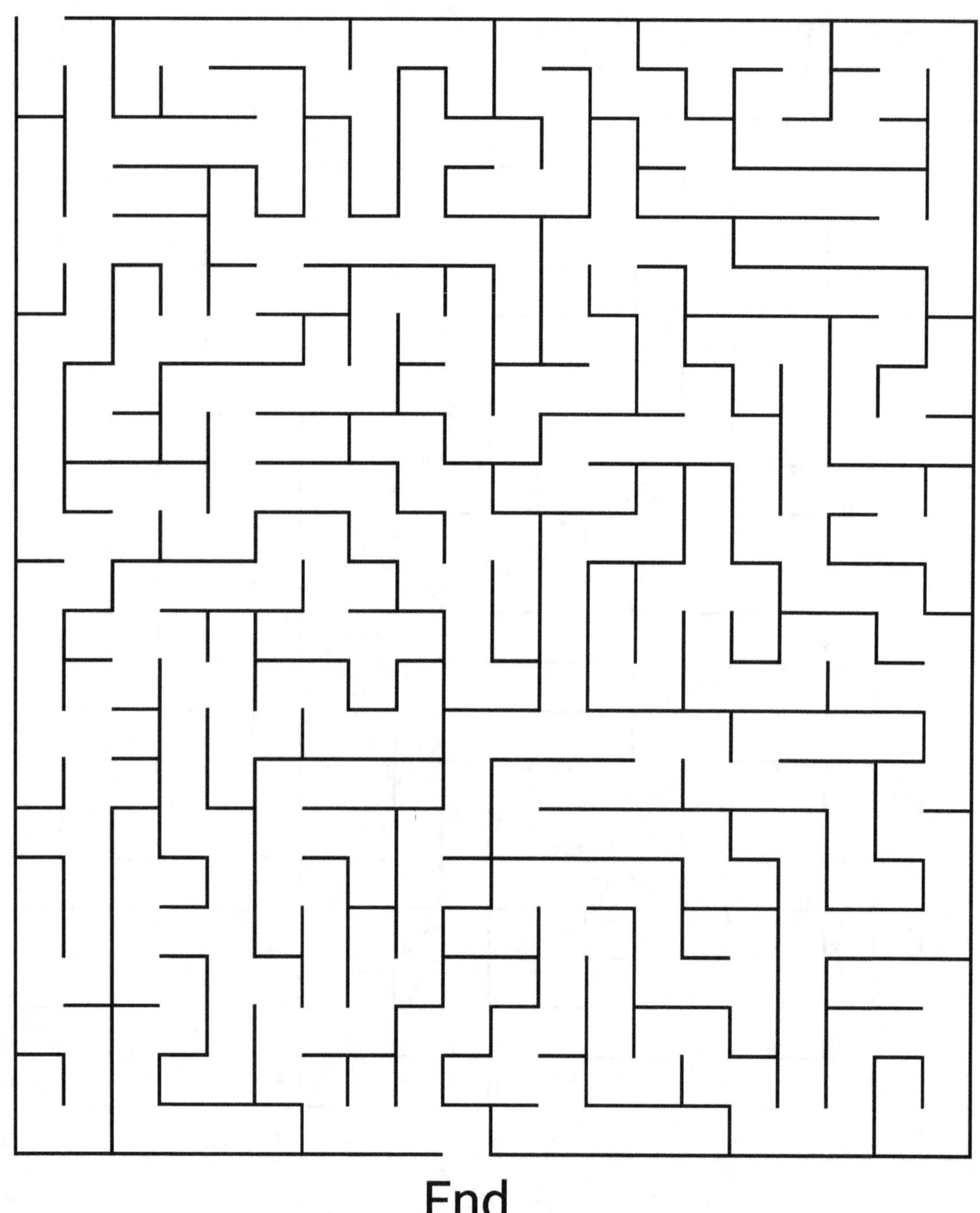

Maze 10

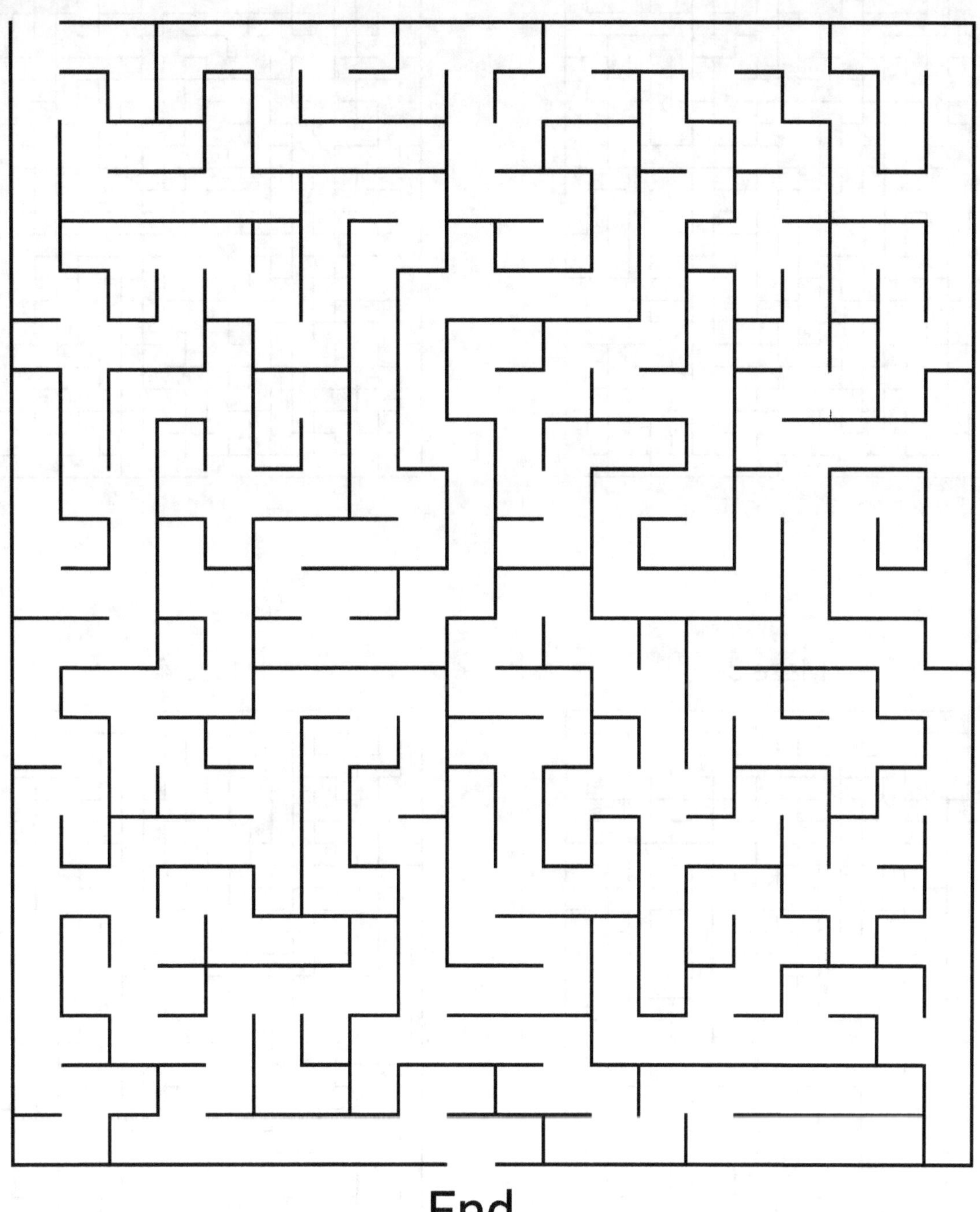

Mazes solutions

Maze 1

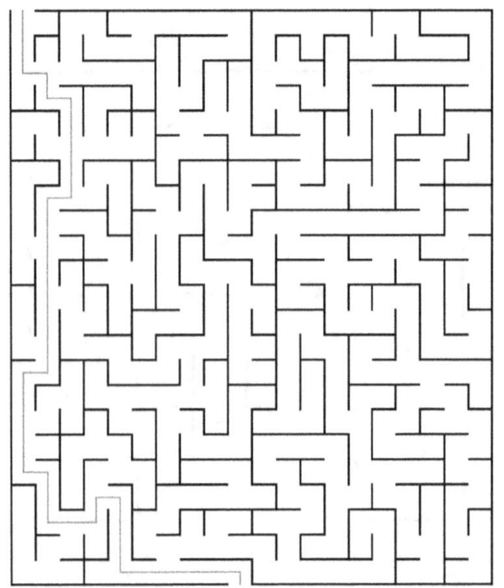

Maze 2

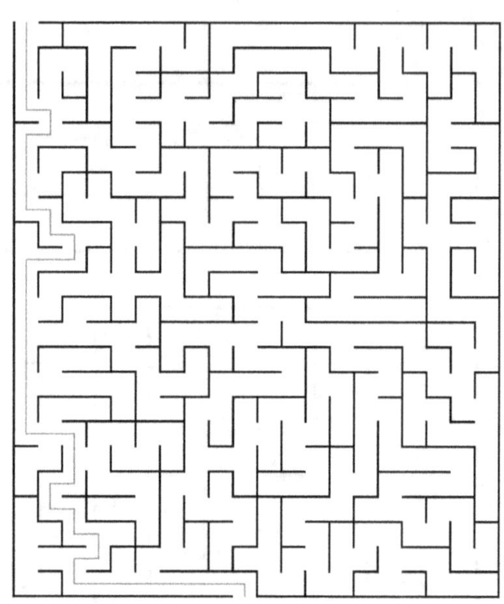

Maze 3

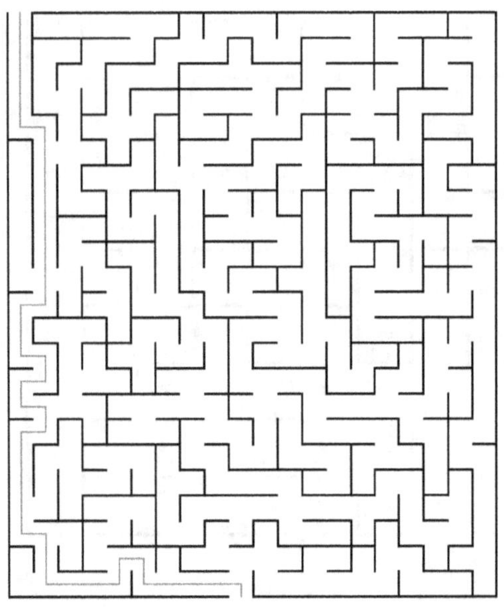

Maze 4

Mazes solutions

Maze 5

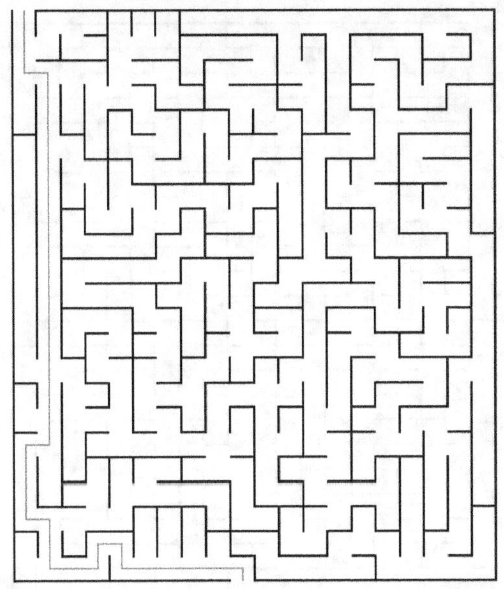

Maze 6

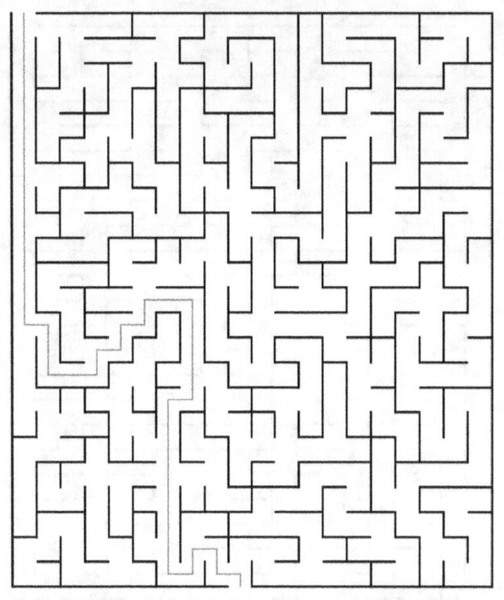

Maze 7

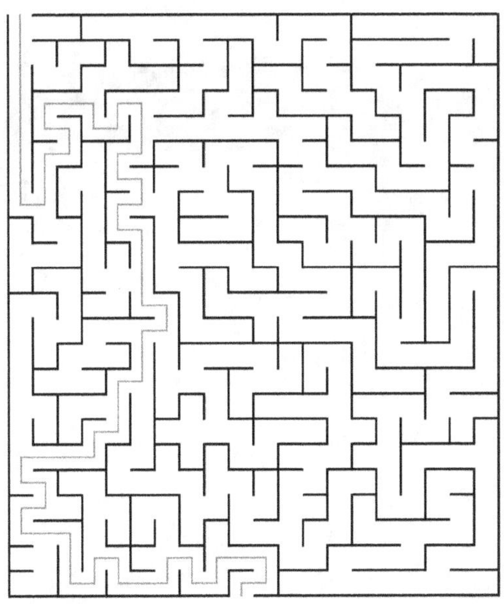

Maze 8

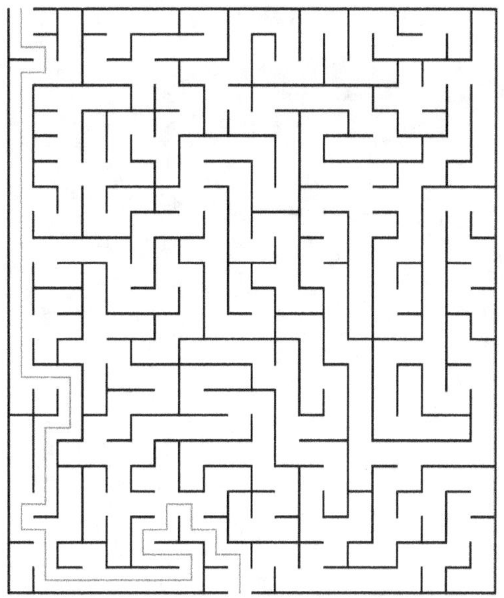

Mazes solutions

Maze 9

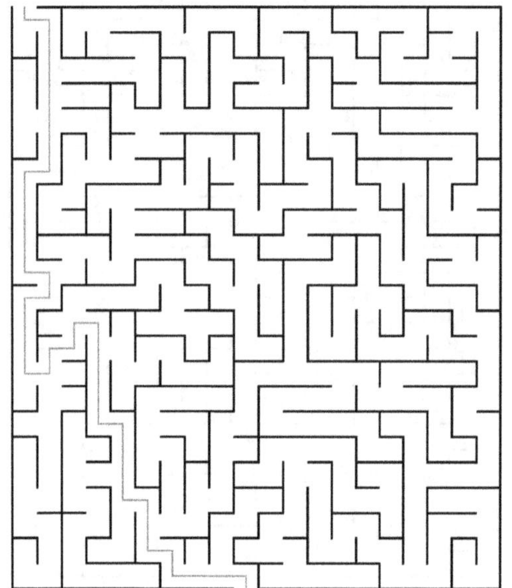

Maze 10

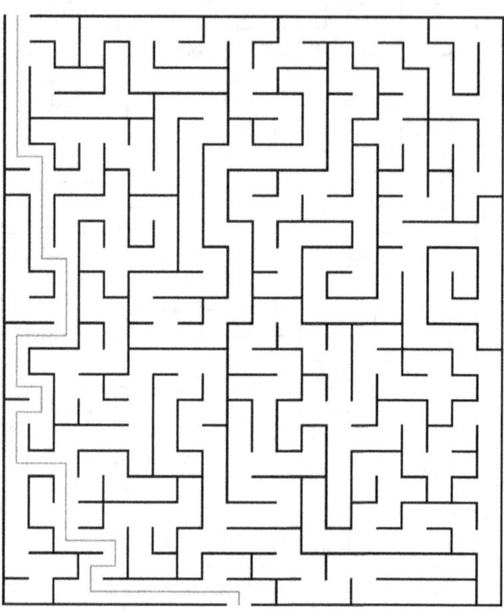

Word Scramble 1

IWHET = _______

DRE = _______

ERGEN = _______

EGRY = _______

EIOVLT = _______

WORNB = _______

NYVA = _______

LNMOE = _______

ABMRE = _______

CCHLOARA = _______

Word List

White	Red	Green
Grey	Violet	Brown
Navy	Lemon	Amber
Charcoal		

Word Scramble 2

ILVEO = ______

BRUY = ______

YIRVO = ______

MDRALEE = ______

BEUL = ______

RUTNBEET = ______

BCKLA = ______

OLEWYL = ______

YKS = ______

LUPREP = ______

Word List

Olive	Ruby	Ivory
Emerald	blue	Brunette
Black	Yellow	Sky
Purple		

Word Scramble 3

NAMGEAT = ________

PNKI = ____

UTESQOIRU = ______

RAGPE = ________

AES = ______

NZREOB = ________

YCNA = ______

ZERAU = ______

TGEANIENR = ________

SPIHPREA = ______

Word List

Magenta   Pink   Turquoise
Grape   Sea   Bronze
Cyan   Azure   Tangerine
Sapphire

Word Scramble 4

EREGN = ________

HAOCM = ______

RENAOG = ______

ELIM = ________

OSINMCR = _______

TADSRUM = _______

CRLAO = ______

TNA = _____

DEERALNV = _______

IGNDOI = ______

Word List

green	Mocha	Orange
Lime	Crimson	Mustard
Coral	Tan	Lavender
Indigo		

Word Scramble 5

ADRK = _______

ERAMC = _______

SLIVER = _______

IMTN = _______

ERRYHC = _______

DOROSOEW = _______

CEOEFF = _______

AHS = _______

OMNROA = _______

MLOSAN = _______

Word List

Dark	Cream	Silver
Mint	Cherry	Rosewood
Coffee	Ash	Maroon
Salmon		

Word Scramble 6

UQAA = _______

CPEHA = _______

RFNFOSA = _______

EALT = _______

BIEEG = _______

FAHUSIC = _______

NDRUUYBG = _______

VMUAE = _______

TRUS = _______

RLPAE = _______

Word List

Aqua	Peach	Saffron
Teal	Beige	Fuchsia
Burgundy	Mauve	Rust
Pearl		

Word Scramble 7

GENART = ________

LCLAI = ________

BURME = ________

LACETJBK = ________

CKHISRWA = ________

LAPERANI = ________

ECBCIYL = ________

KBIE = ________

RAENC = ________

ERRAGCAI = ________

Word List

Garnet Lilac Umber
Jet black Rickshaw Airplane
Bicycle Bike Crane
Carriage

Word Scramble 8

ANV = _______

RRYFE = _____

ICLTOHREPE = ______

AECPJTK = _______

RROLY = _______

ERTOM = ______

WORAPYE = ______

YTOCSO = ______

TCAROTR = ______

TAE = ______

Word List

Van
Jetpack
Ropeway
Eat

Ferry
Lorry
Scooty

Helicopter
Metro
Tractor

Word Scramble 9

UACLNBAEM = ________

ABTO = ________

USB = ________

ACR = ________

EYLCC = ________

GROAC = ________

UCRTK = ________

ODNLAGOS = ________

OOUAHSBTE = ________

LESIMUNOI = ________

Word List

Ambulance	Boat	Bus
Car	Cycle	Cargo
Truck	Gondolas	Houseboat
Limousine		

Word Scramble 10

MCLYTEORCO = ________

ORWBTOA = ________

HIPS = ________

OOERTCS = ________

RTAIN = ________

RNIDK = ________

AEGEL = ________

CCEAKOP = ________

INOEGP = ________

ARKEEAPT = ________

Word List

Motorcycle	Rowboat	Ship
Scooter	Train	Drink
Eagle	Peacock	Pigeon
Parakeet		

Word scramble solutions

Word Scramble 1

IWHET = WHITE

DRE = RED

ERGEN = GREEN

EGRY = GREY

EIOVLT = VIOLET

WORNB = BROWN

NYVA = NAVY

LNMOE = LEMON

ABMRE = AMBER

CCHLOARA = CHARCOAL

Word Scramble 2

ILVEO = OLIVE

BRUY = RUBY

YIRVO = IVORY

MDRALEE = EMERALD

BEUL = BLUE

RUTNBEET = BRUNETTE

BCKLA = BLACK

OLEWYL = YELLOW

YKS = SKY

LUPREP = PURPLE

Word Scramble 3

NAMGEAT = MAGENTA

PNKI = PINK

UTESQOIRU = TURQUOISE

RAGPE = GRAPE

AES = SEA

NZREOB = BRONZE

YCNA = CYAN

ZERAU = AZURE

TGEANIENR = TANGERINE

SPIHPREA = SAPPHIRE

Word Scramble 4

EREGN = GREEN

HAOCM = MOCHA

RENAOG = ORANGE

ELIM = LIME

OSINMCR = CRIMSON

TADSRUM = MUSTARD

CRLAO = CORAL

TNA = TAN

DEERALNV = LAVENDER

IGNDOI = INDIGO

Word scramble solutions

Word Scramble 5

ADRK	=	DARK
ERAMC	=	CREAM
SLIVER	=	SILVER
IMTN	=	MINT
ERRYHC	=	CHERRY
DOROSOEW	=	ROSEWOOD
CEOEFF	=	COFFEE
AHS	=	ASH
OMNROA	=	MAROON
MLOSAN	=	SALMON

Word Scramble 6

UQAA	=	AQUA
CPEHA	=	PEACH
RFNFOSA	=	SAFFRON
EALT	=	TEAL
BIEEG	=	BEIGE
FAHUSIC	=	FUCHSIA
NDRUUYBG	=	BURGUNDY
VMUAE	=	MAUVE
TRUS	=	RUST
RLPAE	=	PEARL

Word Scramble 7

GENART	=	GARNET
LCLAI	=	LILAC
BURME	=	UMBER
LACETJBK	=	JET BLACK
CKHISRWA	=	RICKSHAW
LAPERANI	=	AIRPLANE
ECBCIYL	=	BICYCLE
KBIE	=	BIKE
RAENC	=	CRANE
ERRAGCAI	=	CARRIAGE

Word Scramble 8

ANV	=	VAN
RRYFE	=	FERRY
ICLTOHREPE	=	HELICOPTER
AECPJTK	=	JETPACK
RROLY	=	LORRY
ERTOM	=	METRO
WORAPYE	=	ROPEWAY
YTOCSO	=	SCOOTY
TCAROTR	=	TRACTOR
TAE	=	EAT

Word scramble solutions

Word Scramble 9		Word Scramble 10	
UACLNBAEM = AMBULANCE		MCLYTEORCO = MOTORCYCLE	
ABTO = BOAT		ORWBTOA = ROWBOAT	
USB = BUS		HIPS = SHIP	
ACR = CAR		OOERTCS = SCOOTER	
EYLCC = CYCLE		RTAIN = TRAIN	
GROAC = CARGO		RNIDK = DRINK	
UCRTK = TRUCK		AEGEL = EAGLE	
ODNLAGOS = GONDOLAS		CCEAKOP = PEACOCK	
OOUAHSBTE = HOUSEBOAT		INOEGP = PIGEON	
LESIMUNOI = LIMOUSINE		ARKEEAPT = PARAKEET	

Telling Time

Write the time inside each clock below

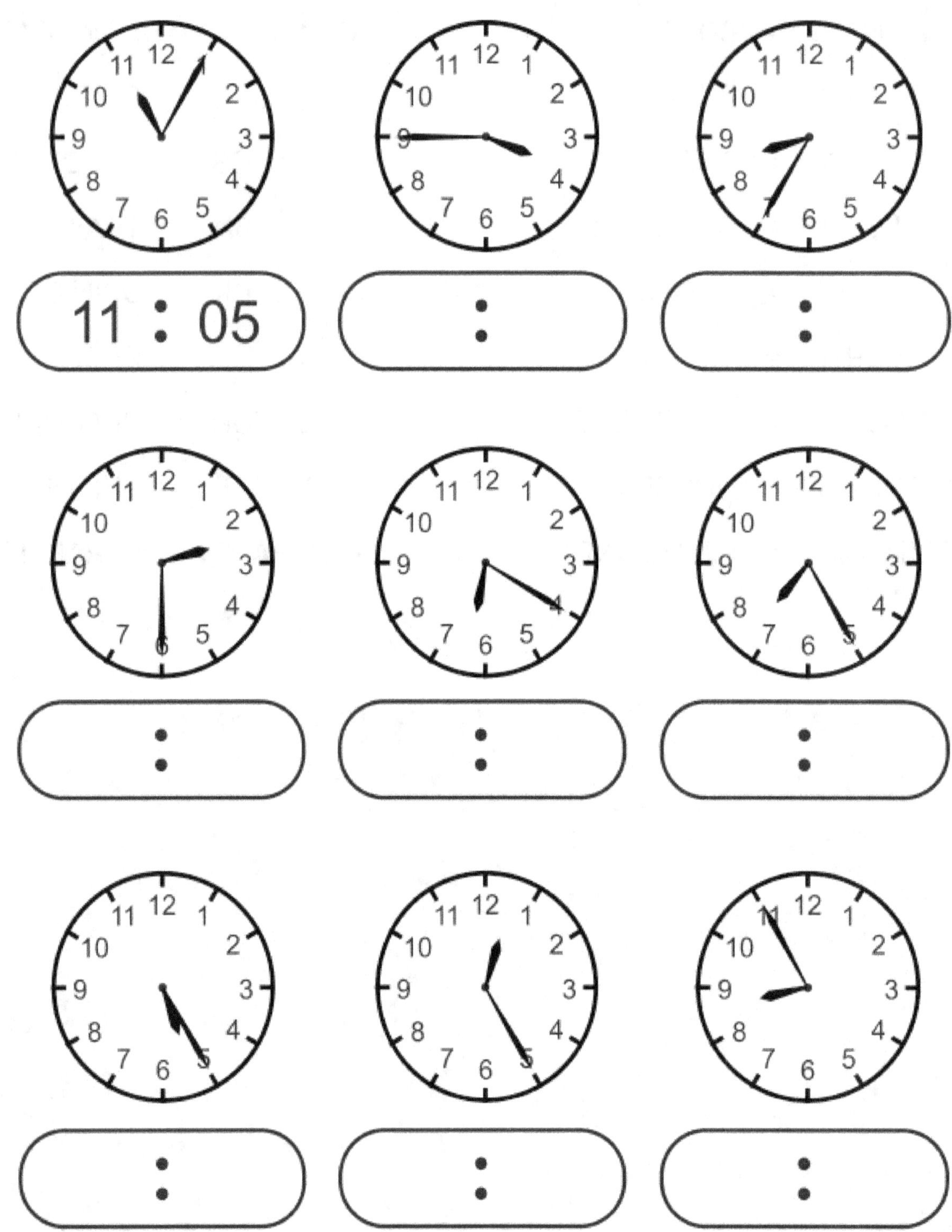

11 : 05

Telling Time

Write the time inside each clock below

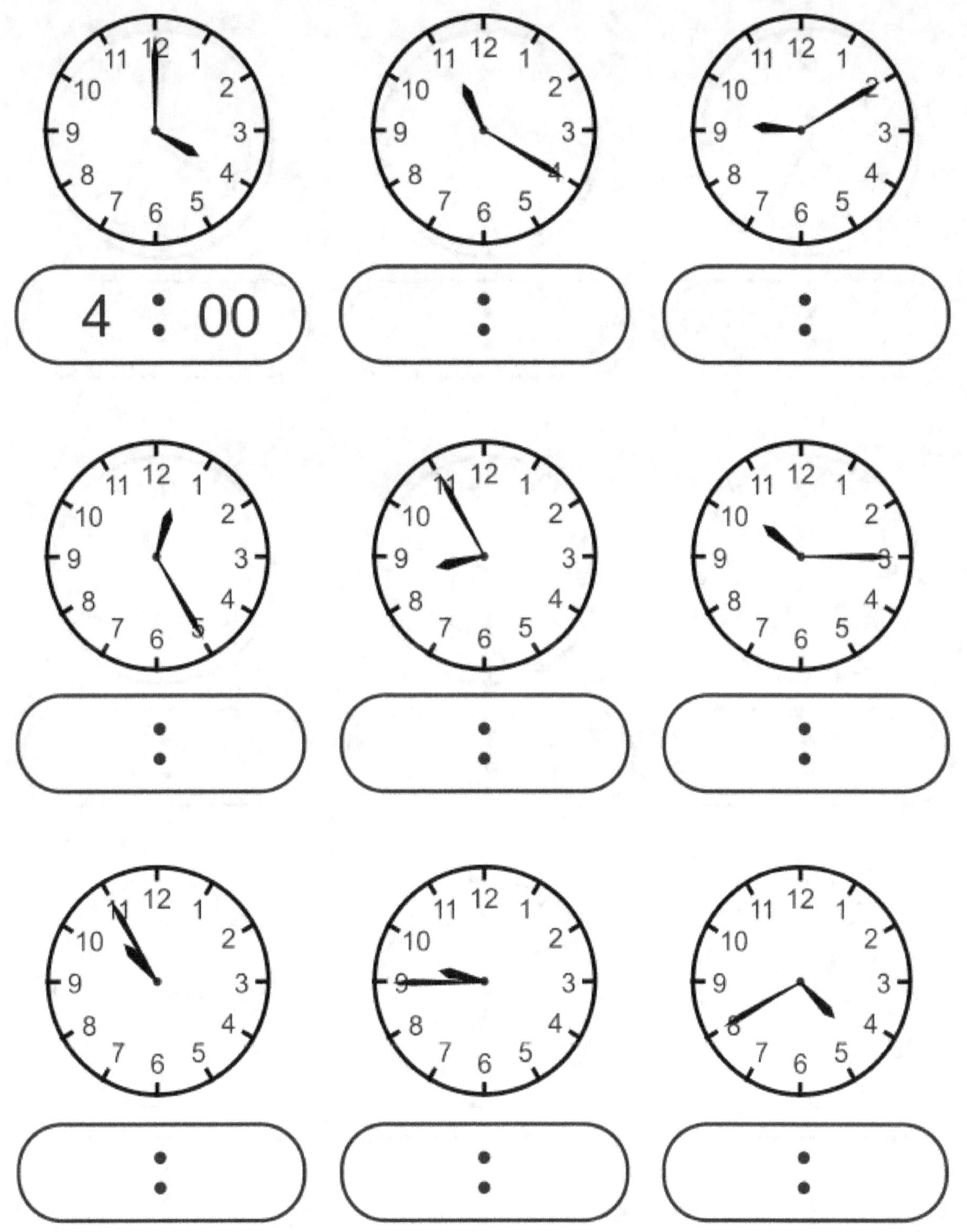

4 : 00

Telling Time

Write the time inside each clock below

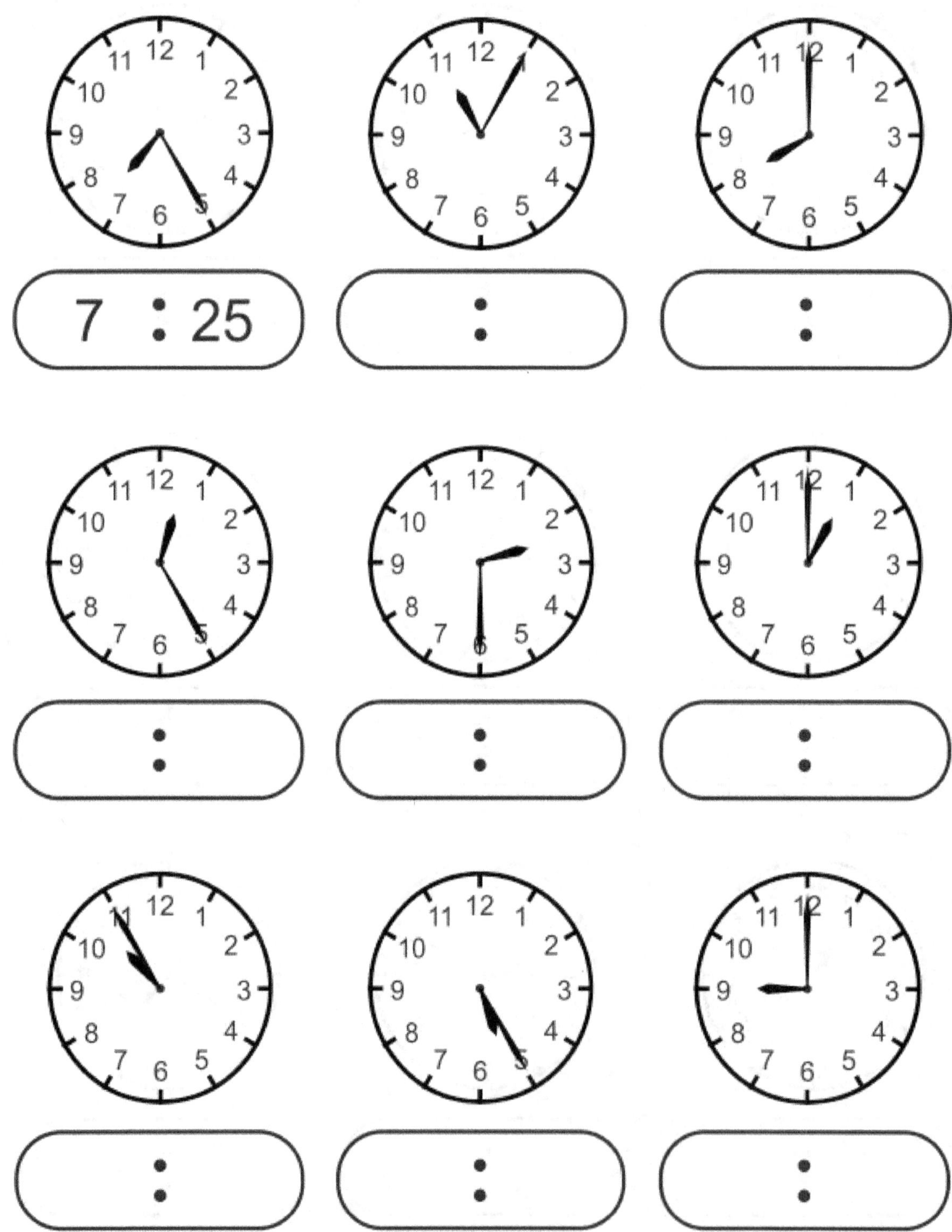

Telling Time

Write the time inside each clock below

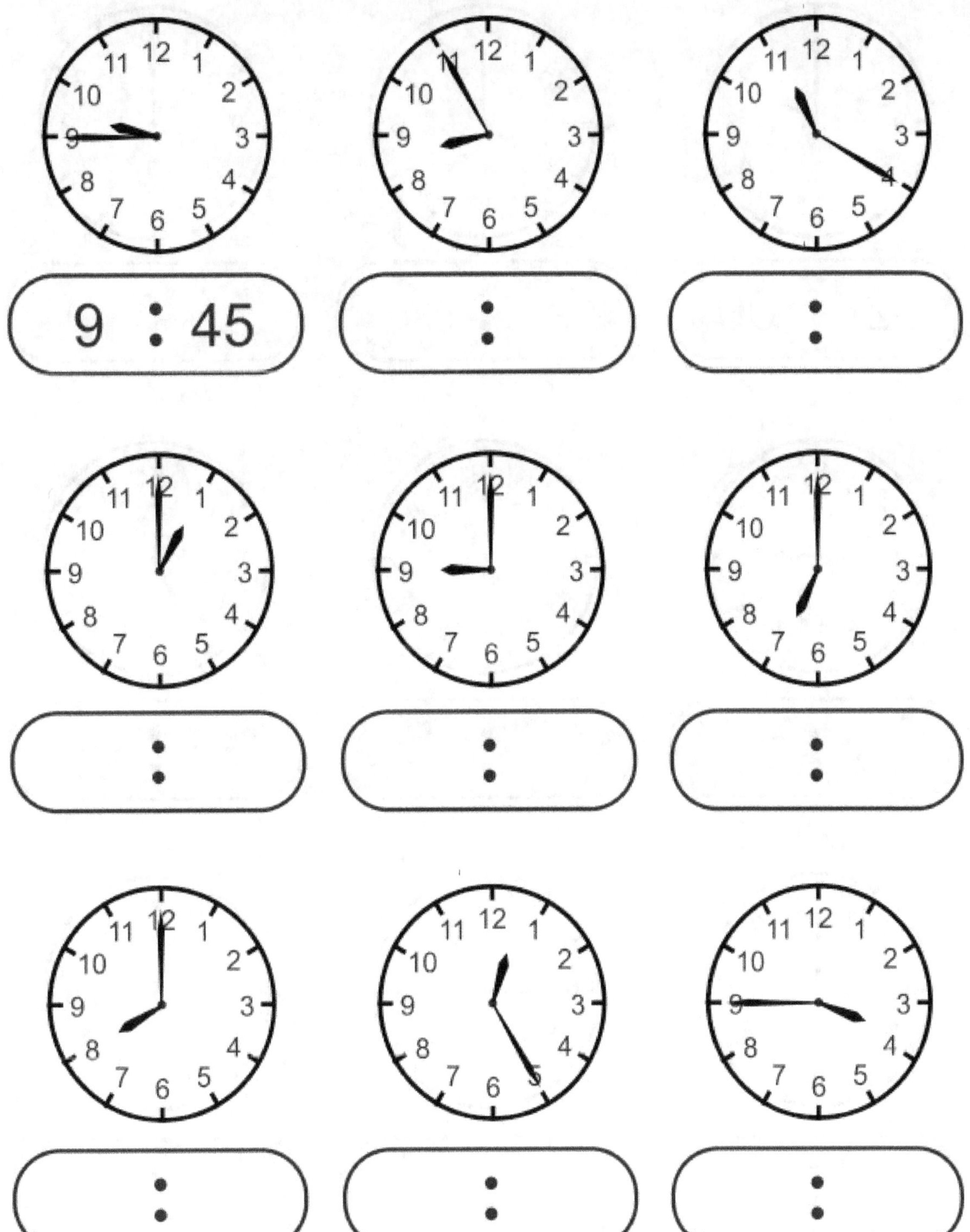

9 : 45

Telling Time

Write the time inside each clock below

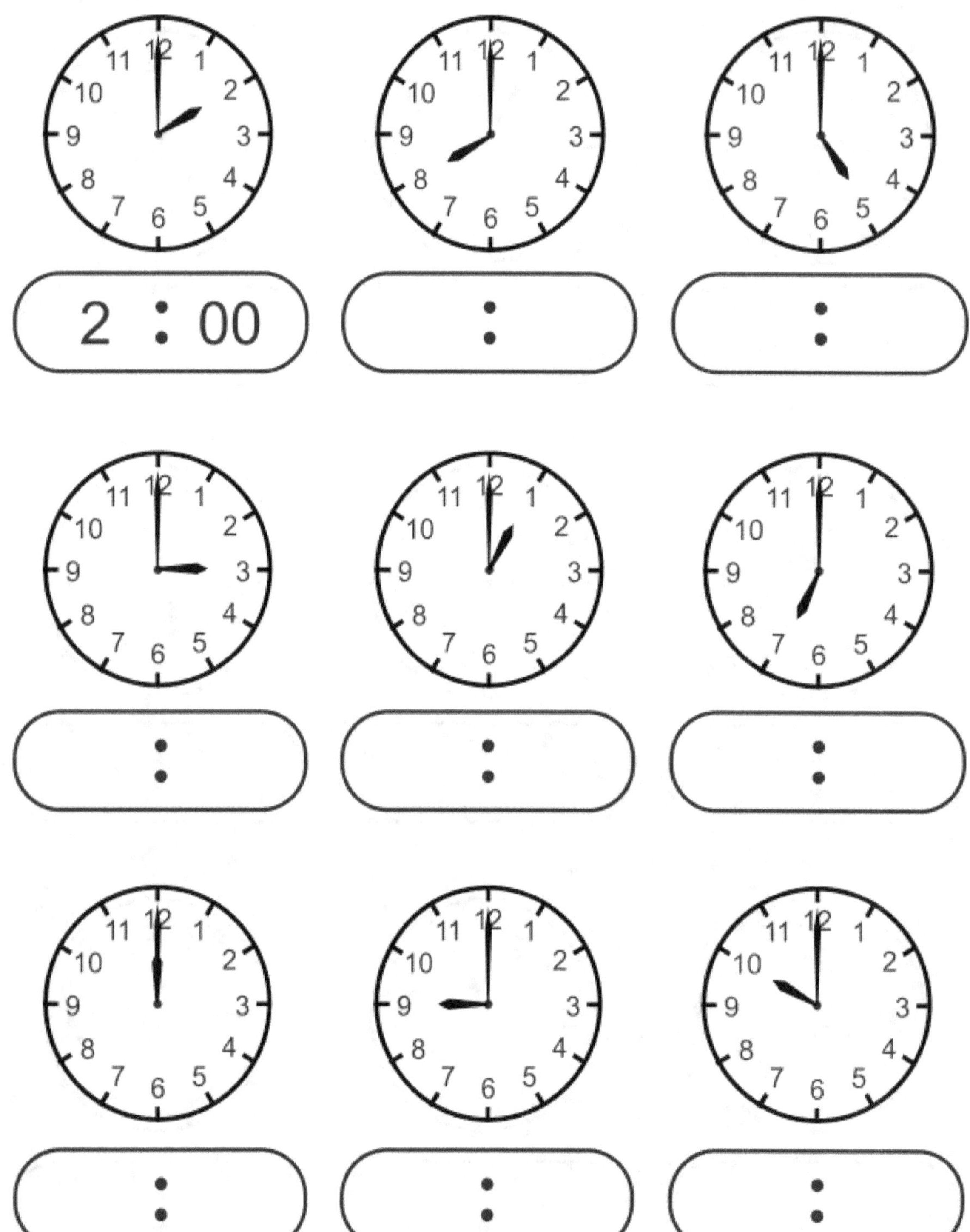

Telling Time

Draw a line to connect the matching times.

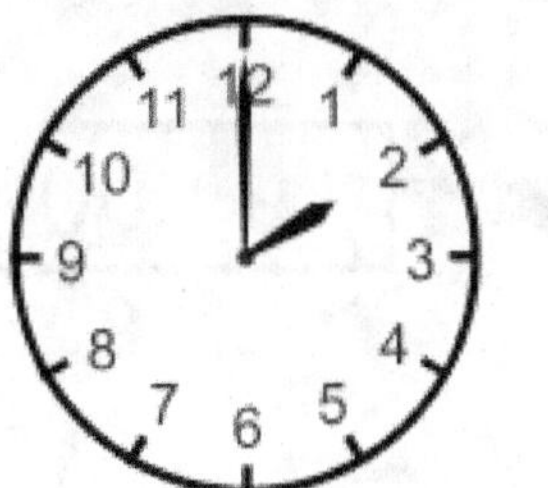 •   • 8 : 00

 •   • 2 : 00

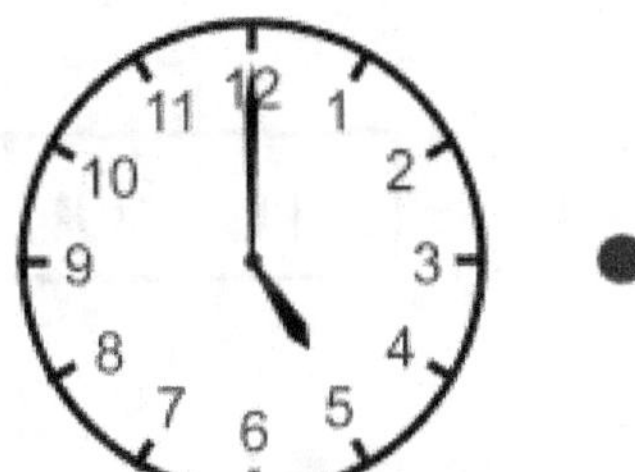 •   • 1 : 00

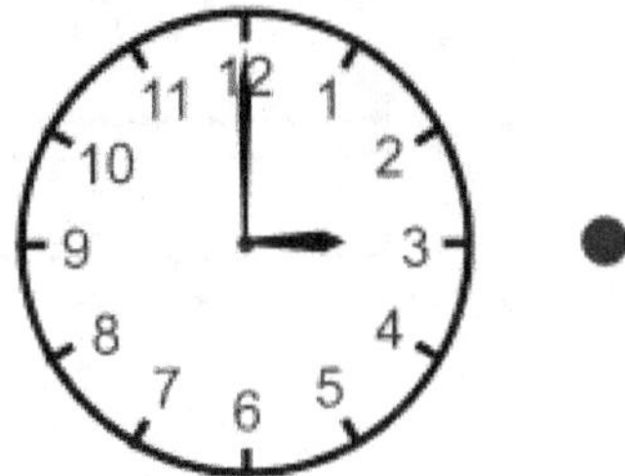 •   • 5 : 00

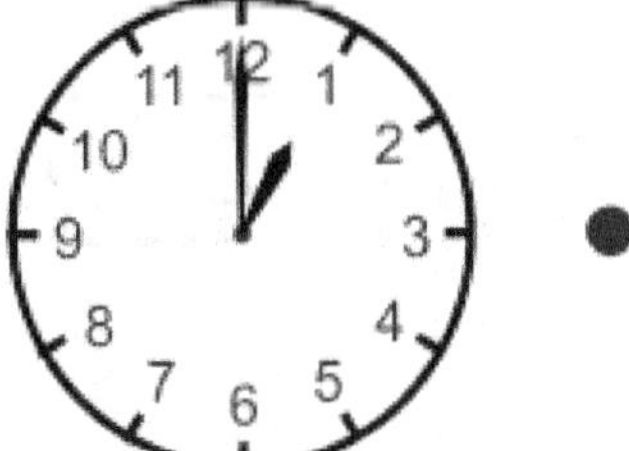 •   • 3 : 00

Telling Time

Draw a line to connect the matching times.

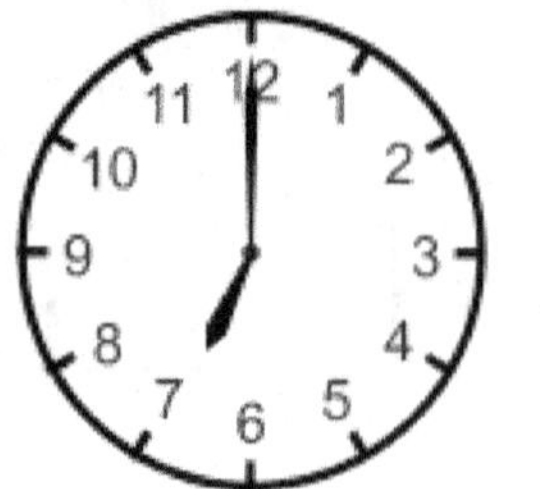 •   • 9 : 00

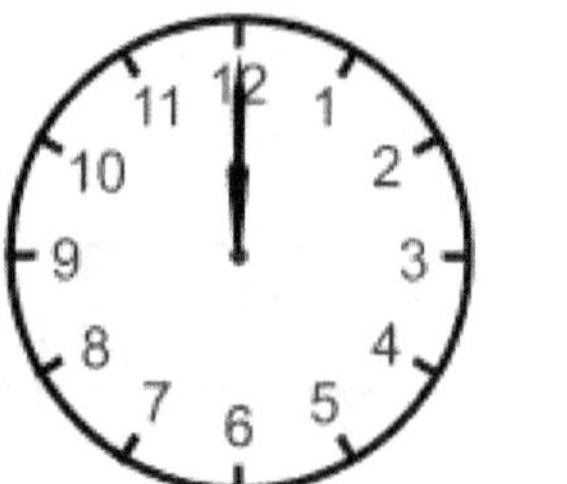 •   • 4 : 00

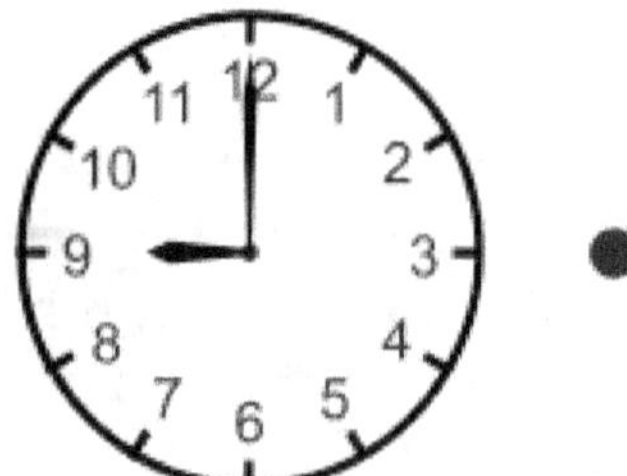 •   • 10 : 00

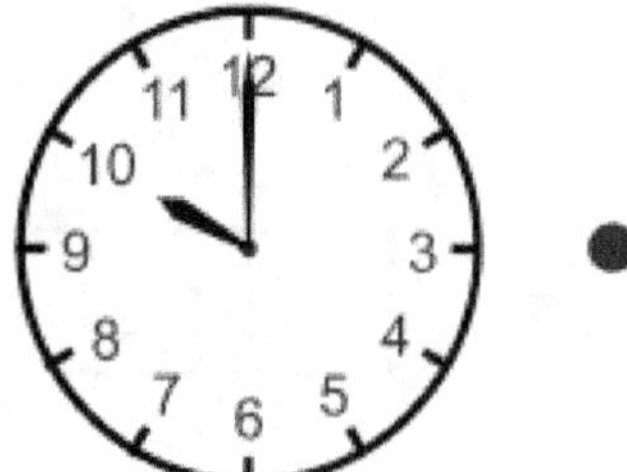 •   • 7 : 00

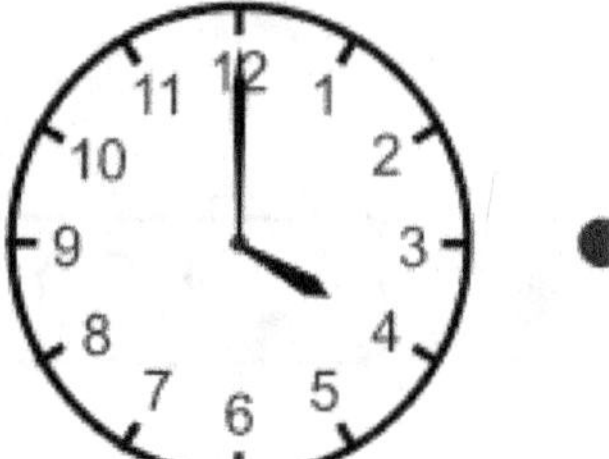 •   • 12 : 00

Sudoku 1

		6	3		
2	1	3			
6				3	
	4	5			
	6		5	4	3
5	3	4		2	6

Sudoku 2

Sudoku 3

			5	1	2
	2				
2			4		3
	4	6		5	
6	1			4	5
5			1		6

Sudoku 4

	1				4
		4		3	1
6	4				5
		1			
4	6		1	2	3
1	2	3			6

Sudoku 5

6				4	5
4			2	3	6
		3			2
5		6	3		
			5		1
2	5		4	6	

Sudoku 6

	3	4			5
6		1			4
4	1				3
			5	6	
5			4		1

Sudoku 7

	6	4			
3			4	6	
5					
				4	
1	5		3	2	
4	2			1	5

Sudoku 8

Sudoku 9

	1	3		5	
	4				3
				4	6
5	6	2	3		
2	5			1	
6					

Sudoku 10

5				6	
	6		5	4	
			3	5	
			4		
	4	6		3	
1		5			4

Sudoku 11

	1				
4		2	1	3	
2	3		5		
		5		4	
3					2
		6	3		

Sudoku 12

		3			6
	1	6		4	
6				3	
	4		2		5
			6		
		2	3	5	

Sudoku 13

Sudoku 14

		4			2
			4		
5				4	3
	4		5	1	6
	6		3		
3			6		

Sudoku 15

Sudoku solutions

Sudoku 1

4	5	6	3	1	2
2	1	3	6	5	4
6	2	1	4	3	5
3	4	5	2	6	1
1	6	2	5	4	3
5	3	4	1	2	6

Sudoku 2

6	3	4	1	5	2
1	2	5	3	4	6
3	6	2	4	1	5
4	5	1	2	6	3
5	4	3	6	2	1
2	1	6	5	3	4

Sudoku 3

4	6	3	5	1	2
1	2	5	6	3	4
2	5	1	4	6	3
3	4	6	2	5	1
6	1	2	3	4	5
5	3	4	1	2	6

Sudoku 4

3	1	6	2	5	4
2	5	4	6	3	1
6	4	2	3	1	5
5	3	1	4	6	2
4	6	5	1	2	3
1	2	3	5	4	6

Sudoku solutions

Sudoku 5

6	3	2	1	4	5
4	1	5	2	3	6
1	4	3	6	5	2
5	2	6	3	1	4
3	6	4	5	2	1
2	5	1	4	6	3

Sudoku 6

2	3	4	6	1	5
6	5	1	3	2	4
3	2	5	1	4	6
4	1	6	2	5	3
1	4	3	5	6	2
5	6	2	4	3	1

Sudoku 7

2	6	4	1	5	3
3	1	5	4	6	2
5	4	1	2	3	6
6	3	2	5	4	1
1	5	6	3	2	4
4	2	3	6	1	5

Sudoku 8

2	6	5	4	1	3
3	1	4	6	2	5
5	2	1	3	6	4
4	3	6	2	5	1
1	4	2	5	3	6
6	5	3	1	4	2

Sudoku solutions

Sudoku 9

6	1	3	4	5	2
5	4	2	1	6	3
2	3	1	5	4	6
4	5	6	2	3	1
3	2	5	6	1	4
1	6	4	3	2	5

Sudoku 10

5	1	4	2	6	3
3	6	2	5	4	1
4	2	1	3	5	6
6	5	3	4	1	2
2	4	6	1	3	5
1	3	5	6	2	4

Sudoku 11

6	1	3	4	5	2
4	5	2	1	3	6
2	3	4	5	6	1
1	6	5	2	4	3
3	4	1	6	2	5
5	2	6	3	1	4

Sudoku 12

4	5	3	1	2	6
2	1	6	5	4	3
6	2	5	4	3	1
3	4	1	2	6	5
5	3	4	6	1	2
1	6	2	3	5	4

Sudoku solutions

Sudoku 13

3	2	1	6	5	4
6	5	4	1	2	3
1	3	5	2	4	6
2	4	6	5	3	1
5	1	3	4	6	2
4	6	2	3	1	5

Sudoku 14

6	5	4	1	3	2
1	3	2	4	6	5
5	1	6	2	4	3
2	4	3	5	1	6
4	6	5	3	2	1
3	2	1	6	5	4

Sudoku 15

6	4	5	1	2	3
2	1	3	5	6	4
1	2	4	3	5	6
3	5	6	4	1	2
5	3	2	6	4	1
4	6	1	2	3	5

Find two same pictures

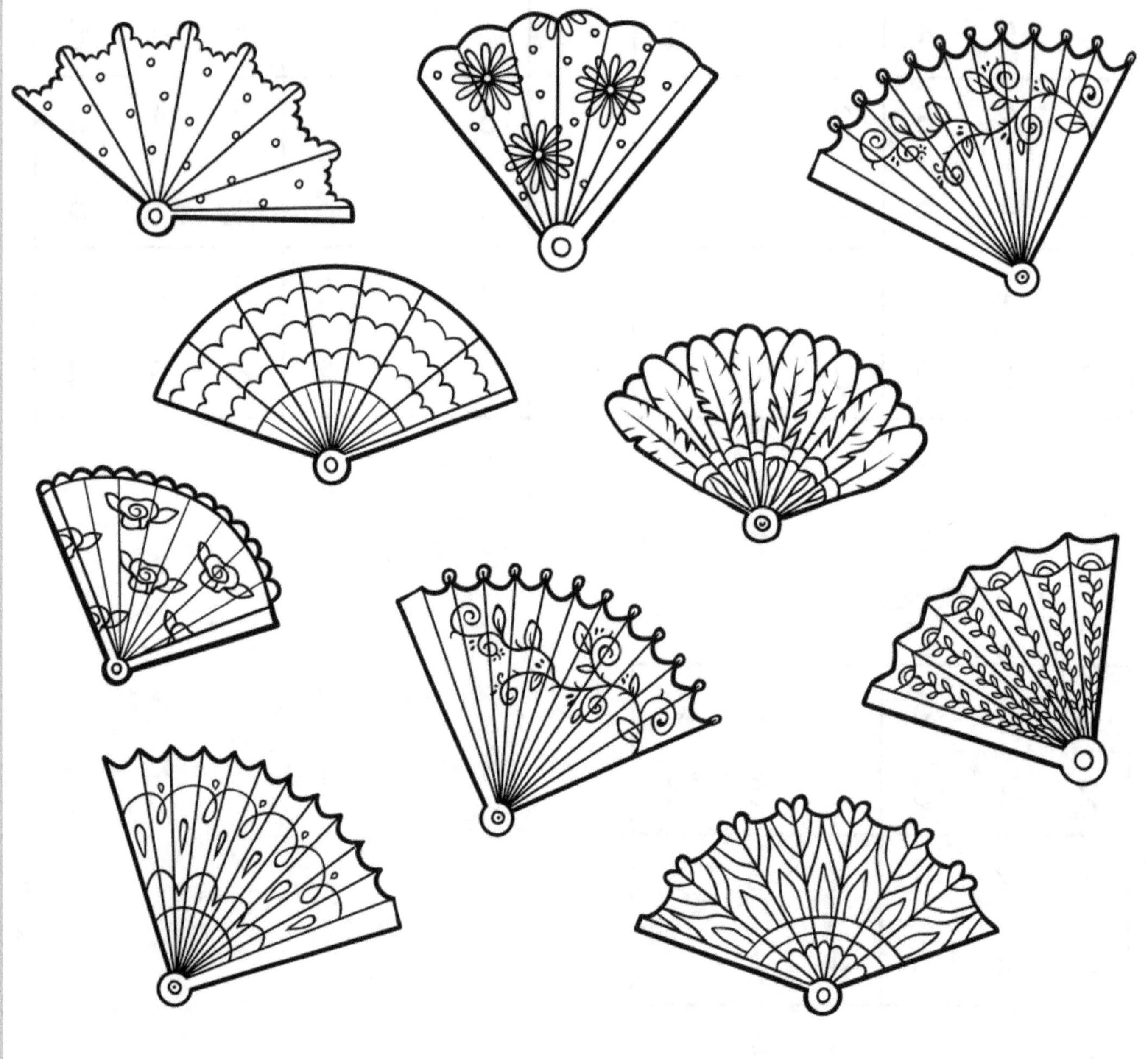

Find two same pictures

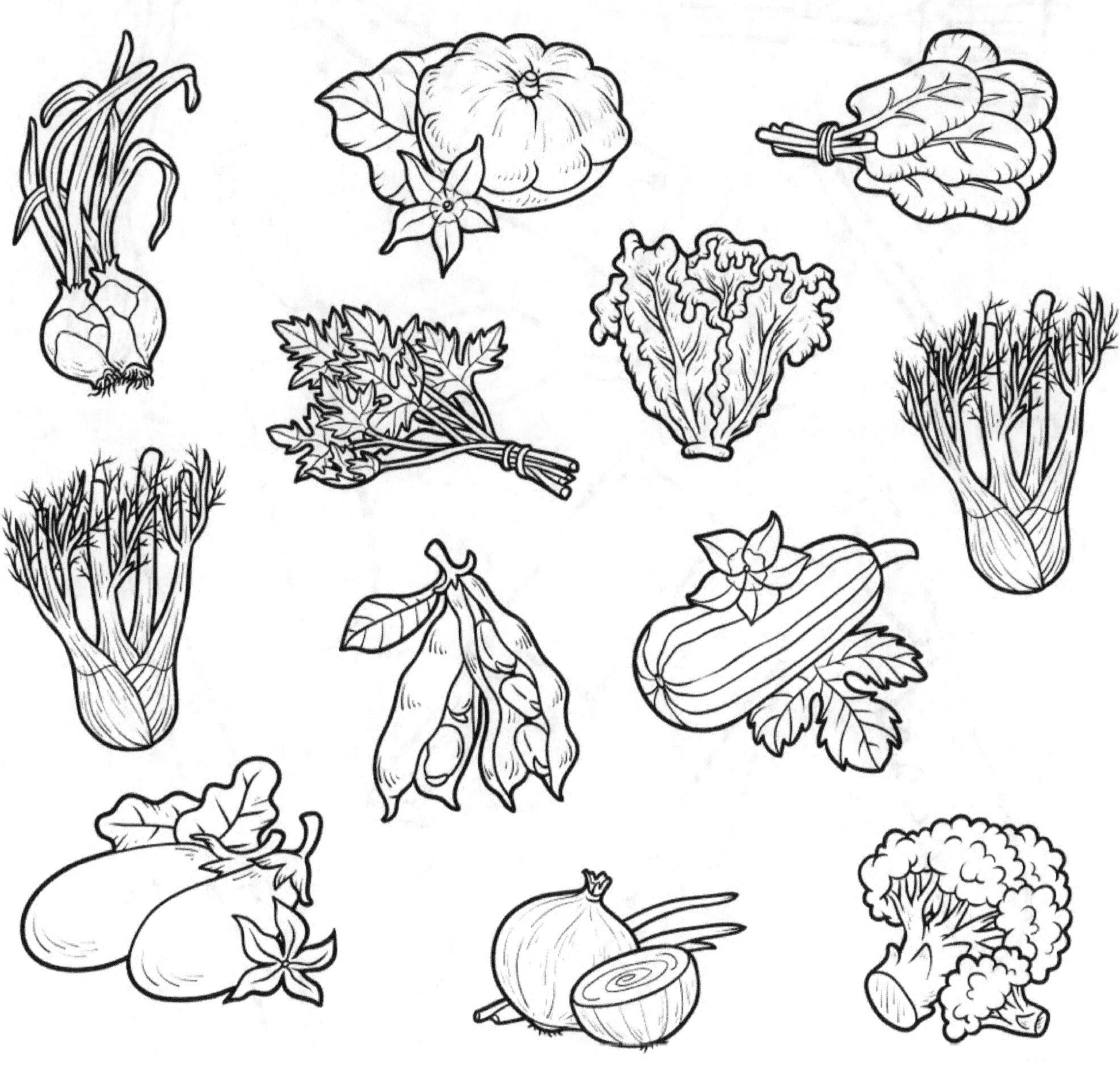

Find two same pictures

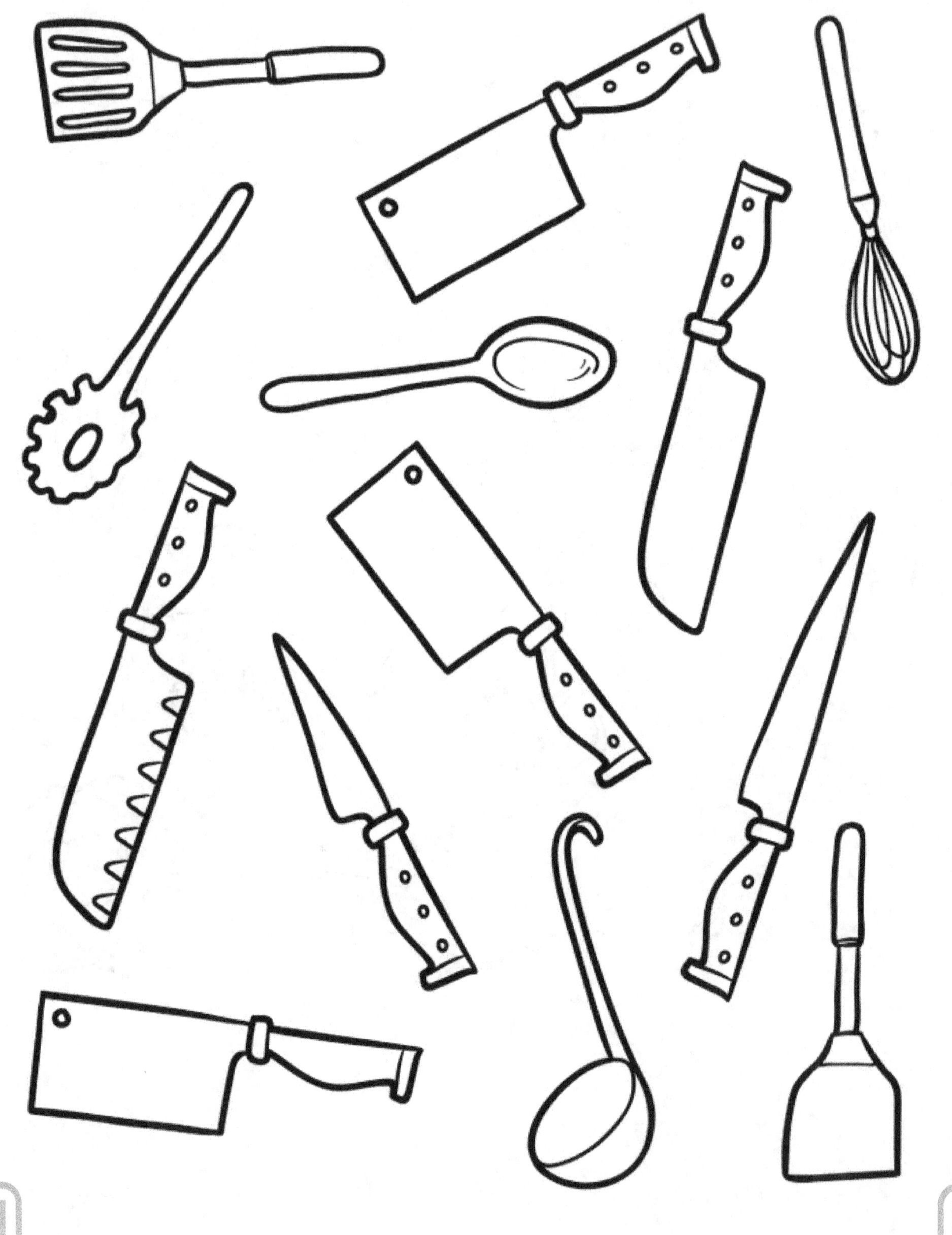

Find two same pictures

Find two same pictures

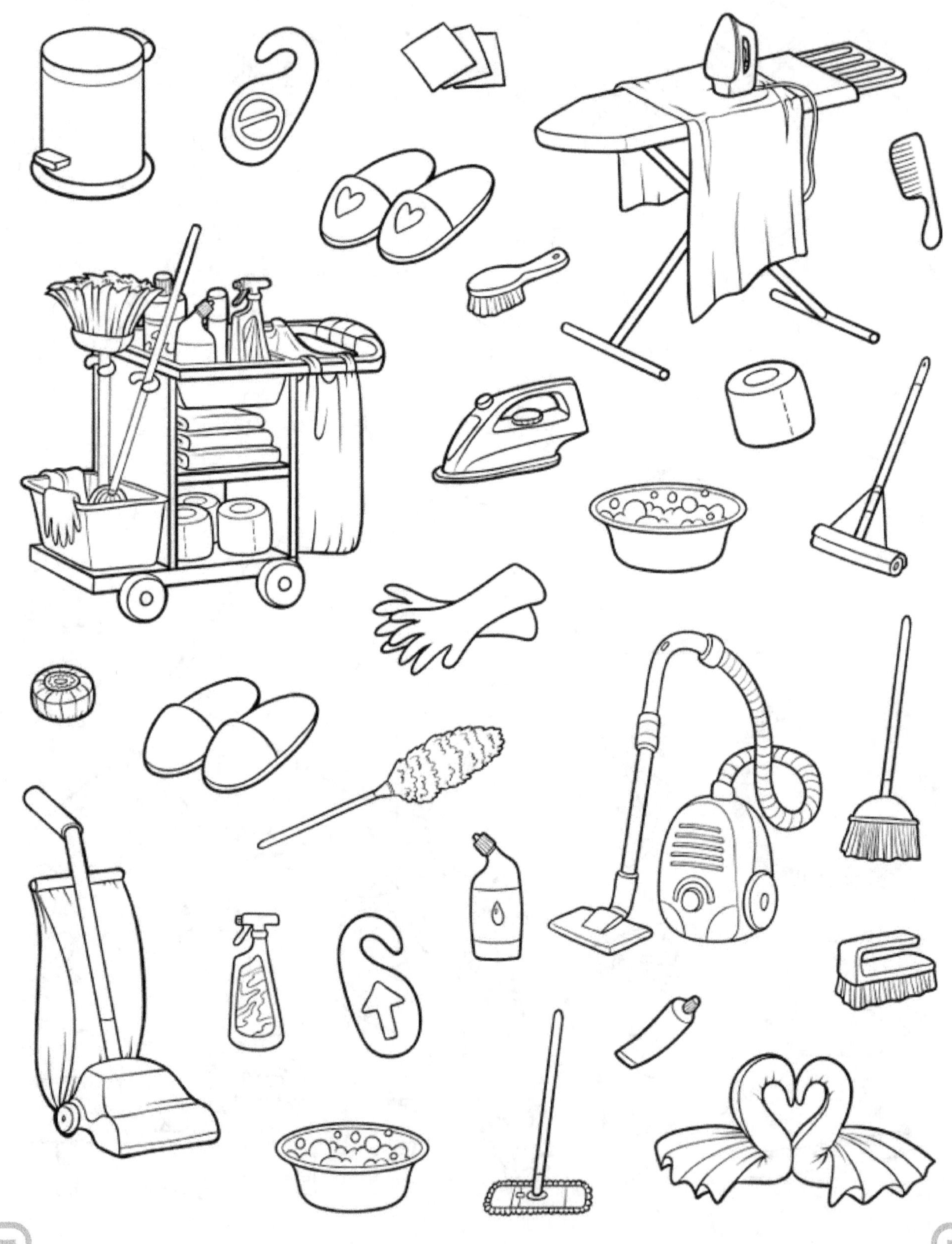

Find two same pictures

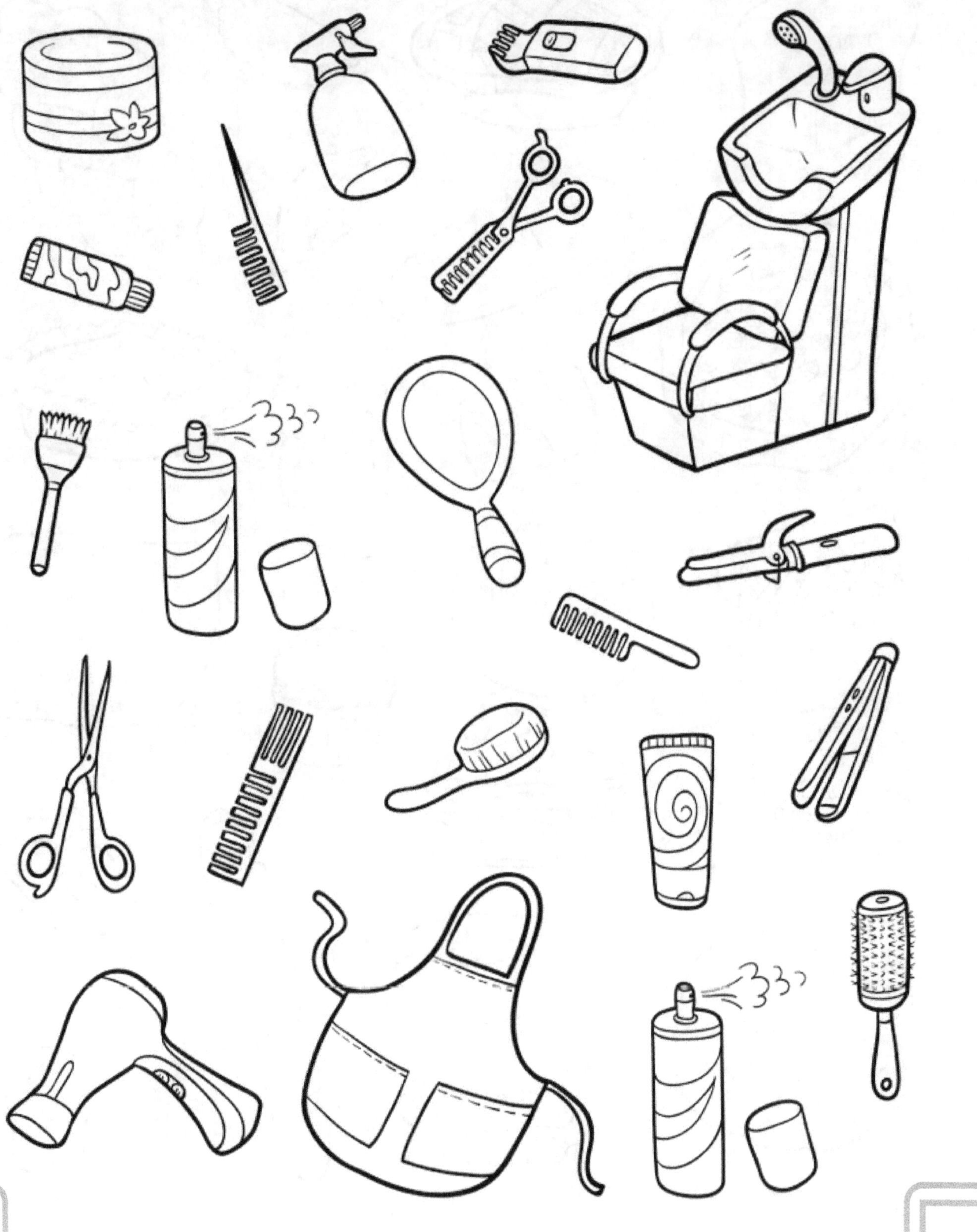

Find two same pictures

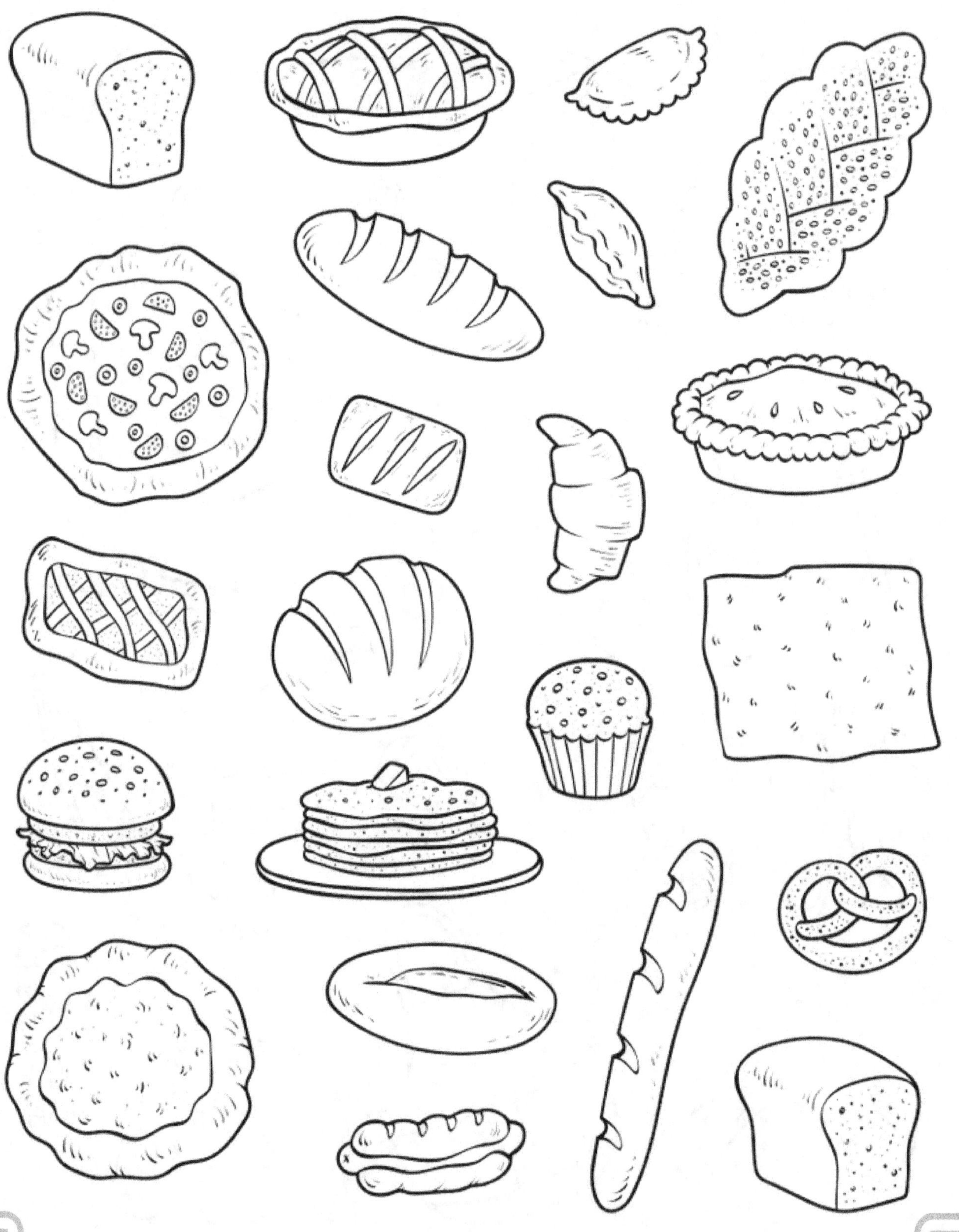

Find two same pictures

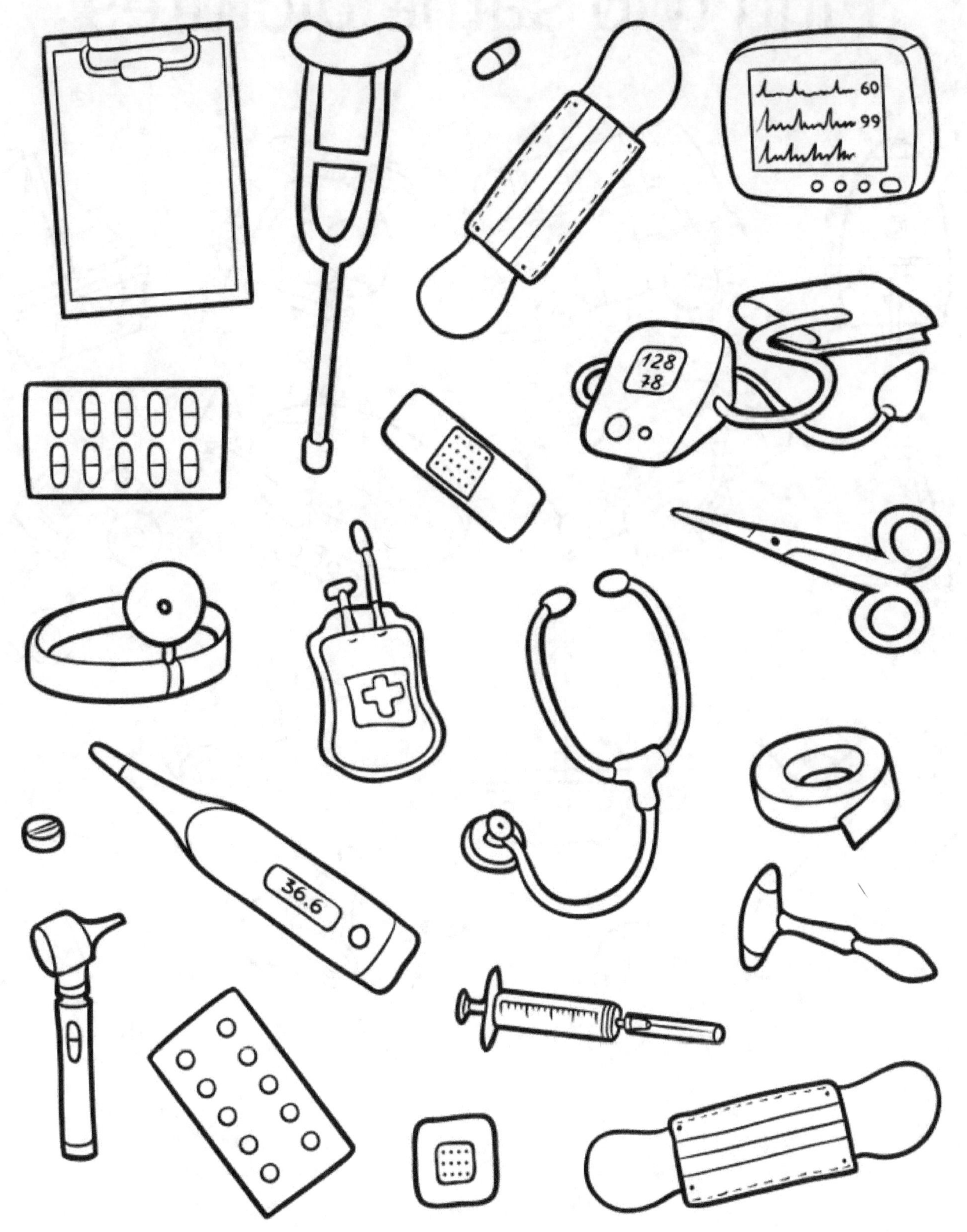

Find two same pictures

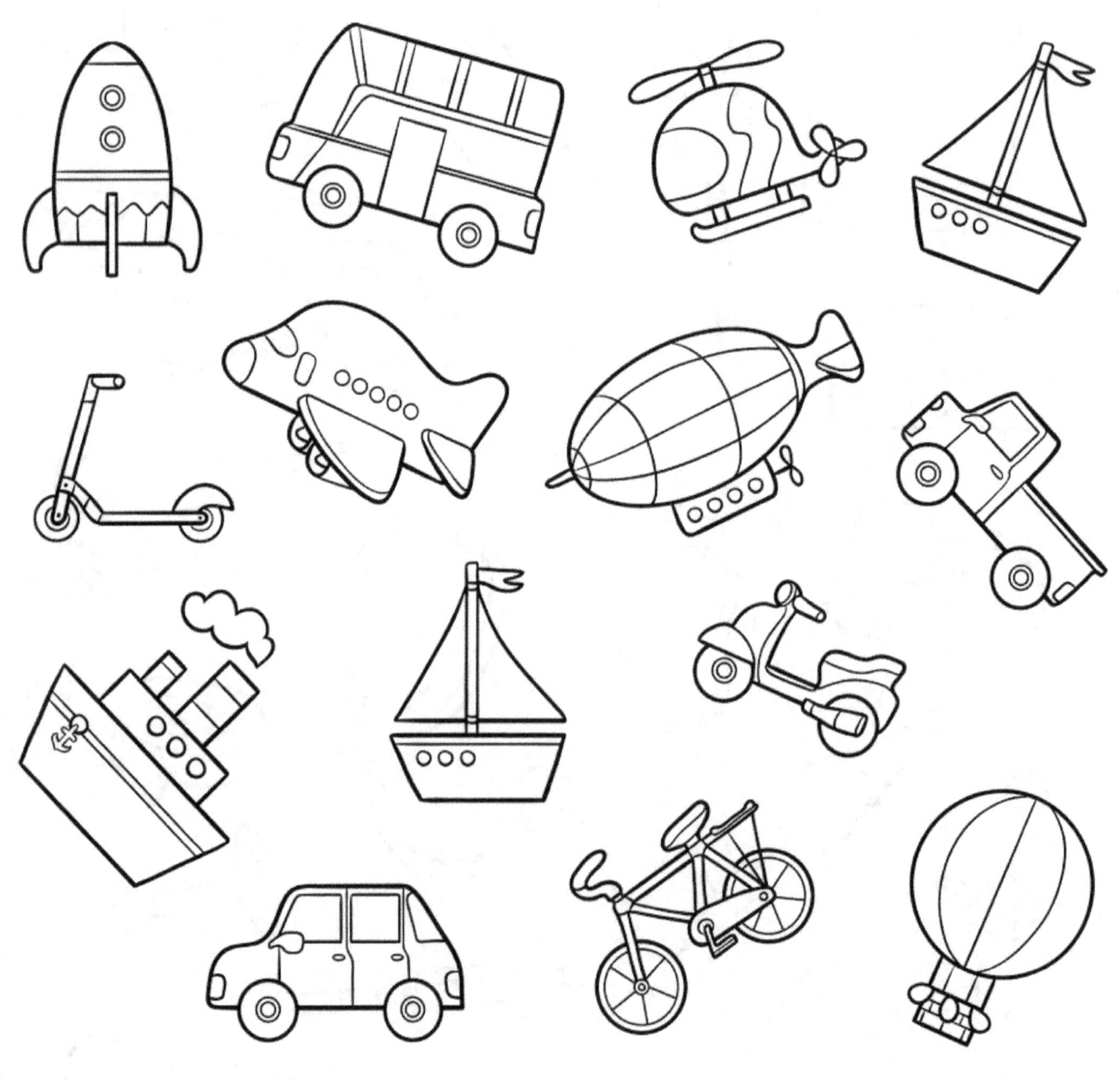

www.ingramcontent.com/pod-product-compliance
Lightning Source LLC
Chambersburg PA
CBHW081219260726
48653CB00010BB/3688